DIAGNOSIS AND TREATMENT OF MYOCARDITIS

Edited by **José Milei** and **Giuseppe Ambrosio**

Diagnosis and Treatment of Myocarditis
http://dx.doi.org/10.5772/46013
Edited by José Milei and Giuseppe Ambrosio

Contributors

Jose Milei, Julián González, Sarah Kantharia, Francisco Salgado, Francisco Azzato, Giuseppe Ambrosio, Rafid Fayadh Al-Aqeedi, Yang, Gerhard K. Wolf, Jordan Rettig, Yoshinori Seko, Andrea Henriques-Pons, Marcelo Villa-Forte Gomes, Marina Deljanin Ilic

Published by InTech

Janeza Trdine 9, 51000 Rijeka, Croatia

Publishing Process Manager Ana Pantar
Technical Editor InTech DTP team
Cover InTech Design team

Additional hard copies can be obtained from orders@intechopen.com

Diagnosis and Treatment of Myocarditis, Edited by José Milei and Giuseppe Ambrosio
p. cm.
ISBN 978-953-51-1082-8

For EU product safety concerns:
IN TECH d.o.o., Prolaz Marije Krucifikse Kozulić 3, 51000 Rijeka, Croatia, info@intechopen.com or visit our website at intechopen.com.

Meet the editors

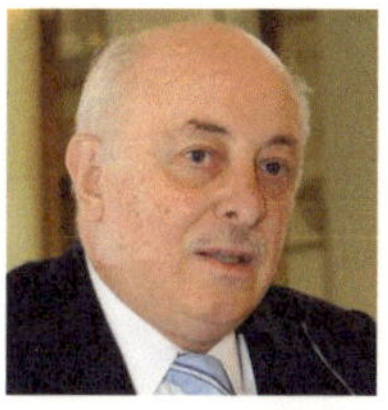

José Milei, Ph.D., M.D., is the Professor of Internal Medicine and Director of the Institute of Cardiological Investigations (ININCA) "Prof. Dr. A. C. Taquini" at the University of Buenos Aires (UBA) and the National Research Council for Science and Technology (CONICET), Argentina. His thesis about the effects of isoproterenol on myocardium was published in Am Heart J in 1976 and has been extensively cited as well as his investigations in the '80 in NIH, National Heart, Lung and Blood Institute, USA under the guidance of his mentor, Victor Ferrans. As a member of the Argentine Society of Cardiology from 1975, he has developed an extensive societary activity. Professor Milei is the Chairman of the Module of Cardiology and Hypertension at the Argentine Medical Association devoted to South American general practitioners´ training. His research on Chagas' cardiomyopathy substantially contributed to the knowledge of its pathophysiology and his work on early atherosclerotic lesions helped set up the basis for the importance of intimal thickenings in plaque genesis. He has authored over 140 papers in peer reviewed journals, 4 books and over 10 invited chapters in books on cardiology. He is a scientific advisor to the University of Buenos Aires and the Director of the Doctoral Department of the Northwest University in Argentina. His work on Chagas' disease has been a reference book in the last 20 years.

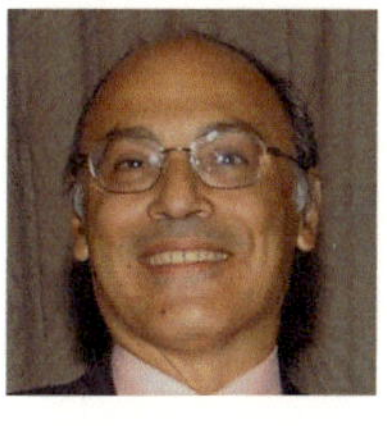

Giuseppe Ambrosio, M.D., Ph.D, is the Professor of Cardiology and the Director of the Division of Cardiology at the University of Perugia in Italy, as well as Professor Honorario at the Instituto de Investigaciones Cardiológicas "Alberto C. Taquini", of the Universidad de Buenos Aires, Argentina.

He has authored over 170 papers in peer-reviewed journals, which have earned over 7,000 citations in international literature and has been invited to give over 70 lectures and seminars at international meetings. He is the member of the editorial boards of many International Journals and an active member of various committees of major International Cardiological Societies.

Contents

Preface

Myocarditis is a clinical syndrome, most frequently of infectious etiology, that presents itself with a broad range of relatively non-specific symptoms, and consists of an inflammatory process of the heart with necrosis and degeneration of the myocardium by inflammatory infiltration of immune cells. The infection can cause direct injury of cardiomyocytes as well as immune-mediated destruction of the myocardium, leading to cardiac dysfunction.

In this book, the broad aspects of myocarditis are fully presented by leading international experts. The texts are devoted to both clinical aspects and pathophysiology, and they present comprehensive reviews of the causes of myocarditis, its classification, diagnosis, and treatment, as well as myocarditis in special populations such as pediatric, peripartum and chronic chagasic myocarditis. Mention is made also of diagnostic aspects, especially by cardiac magnetic resonance (CMR) imaging and endomyocardial biopsy. Pathogenesis of myocarditis, regarding pathways and mechanisms activated during viral infection and host immune response, is discussed. The immune-mediated responses operating in myocarditis result from a myriad of etiologies including infectious, autoimmune, myocardial toxins, hypersensitivity reactions and physical agents, although human myocarditis is most frequently caused by viral infection. Among the viral agents, enteroviruses (particularly Coxsackie) and adenovirus are recognized as the major etiologic factor. However, in the past 10 years, parvovirus B19, hepatitis C, and herpes virus 6, have emerged as significant viral pathogens. Persistence of viral infection, myocardial injury, and adverse remodeling can lead to persistent ventricular dysfunction and dilated cardiomyopathy. Furthermore, acute fulminant myocarditis is a life-threatening condition, which requires careful management.

Clinical manifestations of myocarditis are highly variable, ranging from asymptomatic electrocardiographic or echocardiographic abnormalities to acute myocardial infarction-like syndrome, overt congestive heart failure, malignant arrhythmias, cardiogenic shock, and death. On the other hand, myocarditis is occasionally an unrecognized cause of sudden cardiac death.

Despite the development of diagnostic and therapeutic techniques, acute myocarditis continues to be an important cause of morbidity and mortality among children and young adults. To date, there is no specific treatment for this viral infection

Myocarditis is an uncommon but potentially life-threatening syndrome in pediatric patients who may require critical care transport. Patients may suffer from malignant arrhythmias and hemodynamic collapse and may require transport to a center which offers extracorporeal life support. In one of the chapters a brief overview of pediatric myocarditis is provided, with a particular focus on considerations for stabilization and transport in acute fulminant myocarditis.

Peripartum cardiomyopathy has recently been defined as "an idiopathic cardiomyopathy presented by heart failure secondary to left ventricular systolic dysfunction towards the end of pregnancy or in the months following delivery, where no other cause of heart failure is found". Although, the etiology of this disease remains uncertain, overall, there is more evidence to support myocarditis or an autoimmune process as the cause of the disease than for other proposed etiologies.

Because of these various considerations, it is imperative to have adequate diagnostic tools and effective drug armamentarium. Yet, despite a variety of diagnostic methods, the diagnosis of myocarditis is often difficult to establish. The diagnosis requires a high index of suspicion, particularly in children, as it may mimic other common diseases

More refined, but controversial diagnostic modalities include CMR imaging and endomyocardial biopsy. In general, these techniques would not be employed in an acute setting in a non-tertiary care center. CMR has the advantage of being non-invasive; it requires specialty equipment and radiologists familiar with the interpretation of findings. CMR has a unique potential for tissue characterization, particularly with the utilization of T1 and T2 weighted images, can assess 3 markers of tissue injury, namely hyperemia and capillary leakage, necrosis and fibrosis, and intracellular and interstitial edema, and it may help to increase the diagnostic yield of biopsy for detecting myocarditis due to guiding for biopsy sampling.

The routine indication for performing endomyocardial biopsy in myocarditis has long been a matter of debate; nonetheless, it continues to be the "gold standard" for the diagnosis of myocarditis. Accordingly, the Dallas criteria still remain a reference method for establishing diagnosis. The introduction of immunohistochemical techniques and PCR provided new tools for evaluating endomyocardial samples. Although not yet standardized, they have shown to give valuable prognostic and therapeutic information and are routine testing in myocarditis.

Viral serological analyses in suspected myocarditis are still widely used, although their utility remains unproven. The book also presents results in a murine model of viral myocarditis caused by CVB3. The chapter also describes the characteristics of the infiltrating immune effector cells and their mechanism of cytotoxicity, especially the role of perforin with which killer lymphocytes directly injure target cells and the mechanism of infiltrating T-cell activation.

In the last decades, a number of new strategies have emerged in drug development for the treatment of myocarditis and its sequelae, most notably dilated cardiomyopathy. However, there is no specific treatment for this viral infection. Anyhow, as myocarditis can be induced by a number of viruses, rapid and timely pathogen identification is critically important for guiding early and targeted treatments. Certainly, rapid, sensitive and specific detection of a particular virus or even viral subtype in human samples by detection of virus-specific genes would facilitate targeted treatments. This is particularly crucial for those treatments using nucleic acid-based antiviral agents targeting viral RNA. Interferon beta, immunosuppressive therapy, immunoglobulin, adsorptive immune therapy and monoclonal antibodies, have all been proposed as potentially useful treatments and are fully discussed in the chapters.

In the case of Chagas myocarditis, nifurtimox and benznidazole have been widely used; their therapeutic efficacy varies according to the phase of the disease (acute or chronic), duration of treatment, patient age and geographical area of original infection. The best results are obtained with recently infected patients, when cure rates of 60 to 80% can be achieved, as opposed to the chronic phase, depending on the severity of cardiac dysfunction.

As shown, this book presents a broad spectrum of new aspects of Myocarditis, and we hope it will be useful to general practitioners, internists and cardiologists.

Prof. Dr. José Milei
Director of Instituto de Investigaciones Cardiológicas
"Prof. Dr. Alberto C. Taquini"- UBA- CONICET (ININCA), Buenos Aires, Argentina

Prof. Giuseppe Ambrosio
Professor of Cardiology and the Director of the Division of Cardiology,
University of Perugia, Italy
Honorary Professor at the Instituto de Investigaciones Cardiológicas
"Prof. Dr. Alberto C. Taquini",
Universidad de Buenos Aires, Argentina.

Section 1

Clinical Aspects

Chapter 1

Clinical Presentation

Rafid Fayadh Al-Aqeedi

Additional information is available at the end of the chapter

http://dx.doi.org/10.5772/54362

1. Introduction

Myocarditis is a clinical syndrome characterized by inflammation of myocardium and caused by a myriad of etiologies including infectious, autoimmune, myocardial toxins, hypersensitivity reactions and physical agents. Human myocarditis is most frequently caused by viral infection. Ongoing viral infection, myocardial injury, and adverse remodeling can lead to persistent ventricular dysfunction and dilated cardiomyopathy.

The clinical manifestations are highly variable, ranging from asymptomatic electrocardiographic or echocardiographic abnormalities to acute myocardial infarction-like syndrome, overt congestive heart failure, cardiogenic shock, and death. Myocarditis is occasionally the unrecognized culprit in cases of sudden cardiac death. Autopsy series have reported that rates of myocarditis much higher than expected, with overt clinical manifestation from different etiological agents. Postmortem data have implicated myocarditis in 8.6 % to 12 % of sudden cardiac death of young adults [1,2]. Furthermore, it has been identified as a cause of dilated cardiomyopathy in 9 % of cases in a large prospective series [3]. The clinical history in patients presented with myocarditis remains essential to encompass a wide variety of etiologies, many of which are infectious [4]. In the past 10 years, however, viruses, including adenovirus, parvovirus B19, hepatitis C, and herpes virus 6, have emerged as significant pathogens [5]. The geographical distribution can be of relevance for some forms of myocarditis. In selected countries, Chagas disease, Lyme myocarditis, acute rheumatic fever, and disorders associated with advanced human immune deficiency virus infection are significant causes. Other less frequent clinicopathological variants in the etiological spectrum are systemic disorders like giant cell myocarditis, cardiac sarcoidosis and eosinophilic myocarditis. Additionally, drugs, vaccinations, toxins, physical agents like radiation, heat stroke and hypothermia can be the key point for some rare clinical diagnoses. Although histological findings remain the gold standard for establishing the diagnosis of myocarditis, low risk patients are often given a presumptive diagnosis if imaging studies and a compatible clinical scenario suggest new-onset cardiomyopathy.

2. Clinicopathological forms

The changing diagnostic criteria, multifaceted classifications, and varying patterns of infectious disease yielded great deal of confusion over the past two decades. The morphologic criteria for the diagnosis of myocarditis by means of endomyocardial biopsy was proposed by the Dallas criteria in 1986, which defined myocarditis as a process characterized by the presence of an inflammatory cell infiltration of the myocardium with necrosis and/or degeneration of myocytes that is not typical of the myocardial injury of ischemic heart disease. The inflammatory cells are typically lymphocytic but may also include eosinophilic, neutrophilic, giant cells, granulomatous, or mixed cellularity infiltration. The amount of inflammation and its distribution may be mild, moderate, or severe, and focal, confluent, or diffuse, respectively. A retrospective study of 112 consecutive patients with biopsy-confirmed myocarditis demonstrated, 55 % lymphocytic; 22 % borderline (inflammatory cellular infiltrate with no evidence of myocyte necrosis); 10 % granulomatous; 6 % giant cell and 6 % eosinophilic form of myocarditis [6]. Viral etiology of myocarditis is thought to be the primary cause in most cases. However, a direct causative relationship remains less well established in many clinical occasions. The majority of these cases are classified as lymphocytic myocarditis.

The Dallas criteria are considered the first attempt to develop standardized histopathological description of biopsy samples from patients presented with myocarditis [7]. However, histopathology alone can be inadequate to identify the presence of active myocarditis. Some clinicians feel that the definition is too narrow, owing to the limitation by variable interpretation, lack of clinical prognostic values, and low sensitivity [8]. A combination of histopathological characteristics and clinical criteria has been proposed in 1991 [9] as an alternative scheme to be utilized in the diagnosis of myocarditis. Histologic evidence of myocarditis was demonstrated in 35 of 348 patients submitted to endomyocardial biopsy over 5 years. Analysis of the histologic findings and clinical course of these patients resulted in a clinicopathological classification of myocarditis in which four clinical subgroups are identified. The first form of myocarditis is *fulminant myocarditis,* which is a less frequent form of presentation. The patients present with acute heart failure and cardiogenic shock up to two weeks after a distinct viral prodromal episode. They have severe cardiovascular compromise and may require mechanical circulatory support. Multiple foci of active myocarditis are typically found. The histopathological finding does not match the clinical phenotypic severity. Ventricular dysfunction often normalizes if patients survive the acute illness [10]. In one series, 14 of 147 patients (10.2 %) with clinical myocarditis presented in a fulminant fashion, with the triad of hemodynamic compromise, rapid onset of symptoms (usually within 2 weeks), and fever [10]. On follow up, 93 % of the original cohorts were alive and transplant free 11 years following initial biopsy, compared with only 45 % in those with more classic forms of acute myocarditis. The second form of myocarditis is *acute myocarditis,* which describes patients who classically presented with a less distinct onset of illness with nonspecific symptoms related to the heart. Viral prodromal episode occurs between 20 and 80 % of the cases, which can be missed by the patient, and thus cannot be relied upon for diagnosis. They present with an established ventricular dysfunction and may respond to immunosuppressive therapy or their condition may progress to dilated cardiomyopathy. In a series of 245 patients with clinically suspected myocarditis, the most common symptoms include fatigue (82 %); dyspnea on exertion (81 %); arrhythmias (55 %, both supraventricular and ventricular); palpitations (49 %); and chest pain at rest (26 %), [11]. The presentation can mimic acute coronary syndromes in view of troponin release, ST segment elevation on electrocardiogram, and segmental wall motion abnormalities on echocardiogram. The third form of myocarditis is *chronic active myocarditis,* which describes the majority of older adult patients with myocarditis. They are also presents with a less distinct onset of illness, often insidious, with symptoms compatible with moderate ventricular dysfunction such as fatigue and dyspnea. Affected patients may initially respond to immunosuppressive therapy but often have clinical and histologic relapses and develop ventricular dysfunction associated with chronic inflammatory changes, and mild to moderate fibrosis on histological study including giant cells. The last form of myocarditis is *chronic persistent myocarditis,* which describes a group of patients, who also present with a less distinct onset of illness, is characterized by a persistent histological infiltrate, often with foci of myocyte necrosis but without ventricular dysfunction, despite other cardiovascular symptoms such as chest pain or palpitation.

The previously depicted four clinicopathological forms of myocarditis are still used to describe the clinical presentation and its progression, particularly in the absence of ongoing histological evaluation. These categories may also provide some prognostic information and may suggest which patients can or cannot benefit from immunosuppressive therapy. A new diagnostic criteria derived from limited data was proposed in 2009. The Lake Louise Consensus Criteria utilizes the cardiac magnetic resonance imaging (CMR) for the diagnosis of myocarditis [12]. CMR enhances the ability to detect myocardial inflammation through noninvasive means, as well as to improve diagnostic accuracy. In these criteria, four major domains are considered when making the diagnosis including, clinical presentation compatible with myocarditis, evidence of new or recent onset myocardial damage, increased T2 signal or delayed enhancement on CMR (compatible with myocardial edema and inflammation), and endomyocardial biopsy evidence of myocardial inflammation. Use of CMR appears suitable to identify patients with significant ongoing inflammation, which may be especially important for patients with recurrent or persisting symptoms and in patients with new onset heart failure. The awareness came out that the recommendations proposed by these criteria are based on limited data and that not all centers will be able to apply all components of the suggested protocol.

3. Clinical manifestation

The presentation of myocarditis has a wide range of clinical scenarios, from subtle to devastating, that contributes to difficulties in the diagnosis and classification of this disorder. There are few population-based, epidemiologic studies which have defined the presenting symptoms of acute myocarditis; this is due to the absence of a safe and sensitive noninvasive test that can confirm the diagnosis. Worldwide, the true frequency of disease in its less severe forms, whether clinical or subclinical, across various age segments of the population is more difficult to appreciate. Table 1 summarizes the most significant clinical manifestations and physical findings in patients presented with myocarditis. Typically, myocarditis has a bimodal age distribution in the general population, with the acute presentation more commonly seen in young children and teenagers. In contrast, in the older adult population the presenting symptoms are more subtle and insidious, often with dilated cardiomyopathy and heart failure. Most studies of acute myocarditis reported a slight preponderance in male patients [13]. The male-to-female ratio is 1.5 to 1, which may be related to a protective effect of natural hormone variations on immune responses in women [14]. The variable clinical manifestation of myocarditis in part reflects the variability in histological disease severity. Myocardial inflammation may be focal or diffuse, involving any or all cardiac chambers. Severe, diffuse myocarditis can result in a clinical manifestation of acute dilated cardiomyopathy.

Many patients with myocarditis present with a nonspecific illness characterized by fatigue, mild dyspnea, and myalgias. Most cases of viral myocarditis are subclinical; therefore, the patient infrequently seeks medical attention during acute illness. These subclinical cases may have transient electrocardiographic abnormalities. The reported antecedent viral infection syndrome is highly variable, ranging from 10 % to 80 % of patients with viral myocarditis [15-18]. Appearance of cardiac specific symptoms occurs primarily in the subacute virus clearing phase; therefore, patients commonly present two weeks after the acute viremia. A few patients present acutely with fulminant congestive heart failure secondary to widespread myocardial involvement. Animal models have led to a much greater understanding of the fulminant clinical course of myocarditis, in which rapid progression, severe ventricular dysfunction and cardiovascular collapse occurs [19]. Fulminant myocarditis, manifested by severe hemodynamic compromise requiring high dose vasopressor support or mechanical circulatory support, was identified in 15 of 147 patients (10.2 %) in a large prospective study [10]. Fulminant cases were additionally characterized by a distinct viral prodromal episode, fever, and abrupt onset (generally <3 days) of advanced heart failure symptoms. These patients typically have severe global left ventricular dysfunction and minimally increased left ventricular end diastolic dimensions. Of note, either borderline or active lymphocytic myocarditis can produce this dramatic clinical presentation. The histological features of chronic myocarditis are usually produced a more subtle clinical course. Adults may present with heart failure years after initial index event of myocarditis.

The medical history may embrace a number of hints that merits an emphasis. Previous history of rheumatic heart disease or symptoms defined by Jones criteria, e.g. fever or arthralgia, can be a clue for the clinical diagnosis acute rheumatic fever. History of tick bite may correlate with suspected Lyme disease. Patients treated for neoplastic disorders with chemotherapeutic agents like doxorubicin may draw attention to anthracyclines-induced myocarditis. History of travel to Central or South America can be a clue for the diagnosis of Chagas disease. Additionally, giant-cell myocarditis should be considered in patients with acute dilated cardiomyopathy associated with thymoma, autoimmune disorders, ventricular tachycardia, or high-grade heart block. Furthermore, unusual cause of myocarditis, such as cardiac sarcoidosis, should be suspected in patients who present with chronic heart failure, dilated cardiomyopathy and new ventricular arrhythmias or second-degree or third-degree heart block, or who do not have a response to standard care [20]. In the European Study of the Epidemiology and Treatment of Inflammatory Heart Disease, a 3055 patients with suspected acute or chronic myocarditis were screened, of them 72 % had dyspnea, 32 % had chest pain, and 18 % had arrhythmias [21]. The most important clinical manifestations in patients with myocarditis are as follows:

Clinical Manifestations	
Subclinical presentation (Most cases of viral myocarditis)	
Nonspecific symptoms e.g. fatigue, arthralgias andmyalgias	
Clinical presentation	
	Shortness of breath, orthopnea or paroxysmal nocturnal dyspnea
	Ankle edema
	Chest pain (concomitant pericarditis)
	Palpitation (arrhythmias)
	Presyncope or syncope (atrioventricular block)
	Sudden cardiac death (arrhythmic death)
	Fever
	Flu-like syndrome (e.g. pharyngitis or tonsillitis)
	Thromboembolic symptoms (systemic or pulmonary)
Physical Findings	
	Normal or unremarkable findings
	Relevant physical signs Tachypnea
	Cyanosis
	Elevated jugular venous pressure
	Tachycardia
	Signs of cardiovascular collapse and shock
	Diffuse apex beat and laterally displaced (cardiomegaly)
	Diminished intensity of first heart sound
	Third and fourth heart sound summation gallops
	Murmurs of mitral or tricuspid valves regurgitation
	Pericardial friction rub and effusion (concomitant myopericarditis)
	Bibasilar crackles
	Hepatomegaly
	Ascites
	Peripheral edema

Table 1. The most significant clinical manifestations and physical findings in patient with myocarditis

3.1. Shortness of breath

Dyspnea on exertion and fatigue are common. A history of shortness of breath at rest, orthopnea, ankle edema, or paroxysmal nocturnal dyspnea is suggestive of congestive heart failure.

3.2 Chest pain

Chest pain is usually associated with concomitant pericarditis. Chest discomfort is reported in one third of patients. The pain is most commonly described as a pleuritic, sharp, stabbing precordial pain. It may be substernal and squeezing and, therefore, difficult to distinguish from that typical of ischemic pain. However, myocarditis can be masquerading as an acute coronary syndrome both clinically and on the electrocardiogram, particularly in younger patients [22]. In one series of 34 patients with known normal coronary anatomy presenting with symptoms and electrocardiographic changes consistent with an acute coronary syndrome, 11 (32 %) of the patients were found to have myocarditis on biopsy [23]. Sarda et al., using myocardial indium111-labeled antimyosin antibody and rest thallium imaging, identified 35 of 45 patients (78 %) who presented with acute chest pain, ischemic electrocardiographic abnormalities, and elevated cardiac biomarkers as having diffuse or focal myocarditis. However biopsy verification of actual myocarditis was not undertaken in this series. Complete recovery of left ventricular function occurred at six months in 81 % of these patients [24]. Some presentations of myocarditis, especially those related to parvovirus B19, present like an acute lateral wall myocardial infarction. Ischemia associated with myocarditis may be due to localized inflammation, or occasionally due to coronary artery spasm [25]. It is essential for clinicians to consider acute myocarditis in younger patients who present with acute coronary syndromes when coronary risk factors are absent, electrocardiographic abnormalities extend beyond a single coronary artery territory or global rather than segmental left ventricular dysfunction is evident on echocardiography.

3.3. Palpitation, presyncope or syncope

Palpitation is a common presentation in patient with myocarditis. Presyncope or syncope in a patient with a presentation consistent with myocarditis may be a signal for high-grade atrioventricular block and risk for sudden death. Small focal inflammation in electrically sensitive areas may be the etiology of patients whose initial presentation is sudden death.

3.4. Fever

Fever with or without sweats and chills occurs in 20 % of patients presenting with myocarditis. A history of fever or flu-like syndrome in form of pharyngitis, tonsillitis, or upper respiratory tract infection before admission occurs in 50 % of patients [17].

http://dx.doi.org/10.5772/54362

3.5. Other symptoms

Apart from the nonspecific symptoms recognized like malaise, myalgias and arthralgias, other extracardiac symptoms may identify infectious, toxic agents or autoimmune diseases affecting the heart and resulting in a myocarditis. A viral prodrome of fever, myalgias, and muscle tenderness may precede viral myocarditis, while a delayed hypersensitivity reaction may be first apparent from a cutaneous rash. Rash, fever, peripheral eosinophilia, or a temporal relation with recently initiated medications or the use of multiple medications suggest a possibility of hypersensitivity myocarditis. The clinical diagnosis of myocarditis is challenging, due to its varying presentation and nonspecific symptoms and physical findings. Accordingly, a high level of clinical suspicion is warranted and a presumptive diagnosis is usually made based on patient's demographics and clinical course.

4. Physical examination

The physical examination of patient presenting with myocarditis is frequently normal. Mild cases of patients with myocarditis may appear to have a simple viral syndrome. More acutely ill patients with acute myocarditis have the classical signs of circulatory impairment due to congestive heart failure. Patients may shows signs of fluid overload including elevated jugular venous pressure, bibasilar crackles, hepatomegaly, ascites and peripheral edema. More severe cases may show cardiovascular collapse and signs of shock. In addition to the signs of fluid overload, physical examination may reveal direct evidence of cardiovascular signs in symptomatic patients. Tachypnea and tachycardia are common. Tachycardia is often out of proportion to fever. Cyanosis may occur as well. The apex impulse may be diffuse and laterally displaced suggesting cardiomegaly. Heart auscultation may reveal diminished intensity of first heart sound. The third and occasionally fourth heart sound summation gallops may be noted with impaired ventricular function, particularly when biventricular acute myocardial involvement results in systemic and pulmonary congestion. If the right or left ventricular dilatation is severe, auscultation may reveal murmurs of mitral or tricuspid valves regurgitation. Table 1 summarizes the most significant clinical manifestations and physical findings in patients presenting with myocarditis.

A pericardial friction rub and effusion may become evident in some patients with diffuse inflammation as a result of myopericarditis. Pericardial tamponade was reported in very rare occasions. Pleural friction rub may develop as the inflammatory process involves surrounding structures. In cases where a dilated cardiomyopathy has developed, signs of peripheral or pulmonary thromboembolism may be encountered. Certain physical findings may imply a specific cause of myocarditis. Enlarged lymph nodes might suggest systemic sarcoidosis. A pruritic, maculopapular rash may suggest a hypersensitivity reaction, often to a drug or toxin. Acute rheumatic fever can present with the modified Jones criteria.

5. Electrocardiogram findings

Generally, the Electrocardiogram (ECG) is a sensitive means in myocarditis. However, its diagnostic value is limited by the low specificity and a wide diversity of changes observed during the course of disease. ECG must be timely repeated, since minor abnormalities detected initially may become subsequently more apparent. ECG findings associated with myocarditis may include first-, second- or third-degree atrioventricular block, intraventricular conduction delay (widened QRS complex), bundle branch or fascicular block, reduced R wave height, abnormal Q waves, ST-T segment changes or low voltage. In one report, either ST-segment elevation or T-wave inversion was present as the most sensitive ECG criterion in <50% of patients, even during the first weeks of the disease [26]. A gradual increase in the width of the QRS complex may be a sign of exacerbation of myocarditis. Frequent premature beats, supraventricular tachycardia and atrial fibrillation may arise as well. Arrhythmias such as sinus arrest, ventricular tachycardia, ventricular fibrillation or asystole may occur and threaten the life of patients with myocarditis. Hence, continuous ECG monitoring is crucial to detect potentially fatal arrhythmias.

6. Clinical manifestation of complications

Despite the fact that a substantial number of myocarditis are never coming to medical attention, a less frequent form of myocarditis is fulminant and leads rapidly to cardiovascular collapse and shock that requires mechanical ventilation. In contrast, if these patients survive the first 3-4 weeks of illness they have almost complete recovery and far fewer long term complications compared with those patients with more indolent courses [27,28]. Generally, there are a number of well recognized complications that may be encountered in the variety of clinical scenarios of patients with myocarditis.

6.1. Congestive heart failure

In many patients who develop heart failure, fatigue and decreased exercise capacity are the initial manifestations. However, diffuse, severe myocarditis, if rapid in evolution, can result in acute myocardial failure and cardiogenic shock. Signs of right ventricular failure include increased jugular venous pressure, hepatomegaly, and peripheral edema. The decline in right ventricular function "protects" the left side of the circulation so that signs of left ventricular failure (such as pulmonary congestion) may not be seen. If, however, there is predominant left ventricular involvement, the patient may present with symptoms of pulmonary congestion including dyspnea, orthopnea, pulmonary crackles, and, in severe cases, acute pulmonary edema. Patients with persistent viral genome expression show limited recovery of left ventricular function, decreased stroke volume index and more stiffness of the ventricle with the resultant long-term morbidity of heart failure and a mortality of nearly 25 % [29].

6.2. Arrhythmias

A number of arrhythmias may be seen during the clinical course of myocarditis. Sinus tachycardia is more frequent than serious atrial or ventricular arrhythmias, while palpitations secondary to premature atrial or, more often, ventricular premature complexes are common. Ventricular arrhythmias and variable degree heart blocks are uncommon, but well recognized clinical presentations [30,31]. Persistent complex ventricular arrhythmias after apparent resolution of myocarditis were reported in children and young adults as well [32]. Several series have examined the frequency of myocarditis among patients evaluated for life threatening ventricular arrhythmias that occurred in the absence of structural heart disease [33-35]. These patients tend to be younger than 50 years and to have normal or near-normal left ventricular systolic function. The frequency of syncope or cardiac arrest as reported has ranged from 8 % to 61 % [33,34]. Biopsy evidence of myocarditis among patients without structural heart disease has ranged from 8 % to 50 %. On the other hand, patients with ventricular arrhythmias due to lymphocytic or granulomatous myocarditis have a higher risk. Sustained ventricular tachycardia or new heart block in the setting of rapidly progressive congestive heart failure suggests giant cell myocarditis.

Granulomatous myocarditis has been associated more frequently with life threatening ventricular arrhythmias, syncope, and high-grade atrioventricular block requiring temporary or permanent ventricular pacing than has lymphocytic myocarditis [36-38]. Furthermore, granulomatous myocarditis might be suspected in patients who present with apparently chronic dilated cardiomyopathy yet with new ventricular arrhythmias or heart block or who do not have a response to optimal care [20].

6.3. Sudden cardiac death

The risk of sudden arrhythmic death in patients with myocarditis is increasingly appreciated in the current morbidity and mortality data. The discovery of myocarditis in 1 to 9 % of routine postmortem examinations suggests that myocarditis is a major cause of sudden, unexpected death [16]. Although heart failure and cardiomyopathy are more common clinical presentations, patients with myocarditis may present with syncope or unexpected sudden cardiac death, presumably due to ventricular tachycardia or fibrillation [39-42]. Myocarditis is a significant cause of sudden, unexpected death in adults younger than age 40 years and elite young athletes. In these presumably healthy individuals, autopsy findings have revealed myocarditis in up to 20 % of cases [43]. In an autopsy series of patients under age 40 who presented with sudden death in the absence of known heart disease, myocarditis was responsible for 22 % of cases under age 30 and 11 % in older subjects [39]. In another autopsy study of sudden death occurring in 1866 competitive athletes, myocarditis was present in 6 % of the cardiovascular deaths [44]. In one more series of autopsies in military recruits, myocarditis accounted for 20 % of deaths due to identifiable structural cardiac abnormalities [40].

6.4. Dilated cardiomyopathy

A substantial subset of symptomatic cases of postviral or lymphocytic myocarditis present with a syndrome of heart failure and dilated cardiomyopathy. A clinical and pathologic syndrome that is similar to dilated cardiomyopathy (DCM) may develop after resolution of viral myocarditis in animal models and biopsy-proven myocarditis in human subjects [45]. This has led to speculation that DCM may develop in some individuals as a result of subclinical viral myocarditis. Theoretically, an episode of myocarditis could initiate a variety of autoimmune reactions that injure the myocardium and ultimately result in the development of DCM. These abnormalities in immune regulation and the variety of antimyocardial antibodies present in DCM are consistent with this hypothesis. Enteroviral RNA sequences may be found in heart biopsy samples in DCM but with a very variable frequency (0–30 %), [46,47]. Furthermore, analysis of human viruses other than enteroviruses suggests that adenoviruses, herpes, and cytomegalovirus can also cause myocarditis and potentially DCM, particularly in children and young subjects [48,49].

In most acute cases of lymphocytic myocarditis, left ventricular function improves over one to six months with standard heart failure care. However a substantial minority will develop a persistent inflammation that leads to chronic cardiomyopathy. In the patients who develop chronic cardiomyopathy, the risk of heart transplantation and death is high. In a large review of 1230 cases of initially unexplained cardiomyopathy, 9 % were thought to be due to myocarditis [50]. A similar prevalence of 10 % was noted in the Myocarditis Treatment Trial in which endomyocardial biopsy was performed in over 2200 patients with unexplained heart failure of less than 2 years duration [18].

6.5. Thromboembolism

Thromboembolism, arterial and venous, is more evident in patients with left ventricular dysfunction, and appears to be quite frequent complication in certain forms of myocarditis and cardiomyopathies. Additionally, the risk of thromboembolism from either tissue or thrombus from the biopsy site is higher in left ventricular biopsy. Right-sided thromboembolism can be due to thrombus from the venous access sheath, particularly with the internal jugular approach. The possibility of some small added diagnostic yield by taking biopsy samples of the left ventricle in addition to the right is outweighed by the attendant risk of systemic embolism.

Thromboembolism is frequent in advanced Chagas disease, and its occurrence is probably underestimated [51,52]. At autopsy, 73 % of patients have left or right ventricular mural thrombi, with evidence of pulmonary or systemic embolization in 60 % [53]. The apical aneurysm typical of Chagas disease is particularly prone to the formation of thrombi and is associated with a high incidence of thromboembolic events [54]. Furthermore, there is a high incidence of thromboembolism in population with peripartum cardiomyopathy. Thrombi are the result of the hypercoagulable state of pregnancy and of stasis and turbulent flow in the dilated heart. Thrombi often form in patients with lower left ventricular ejection fraction (<35 %), [55,56]. Higher mortality rates have been reported to be due to thromboembolism as well [57].

6.6. Recurrent myocarditis

In the majority of patients, the clinical course of myocarditis is self-limited, and there is complete resolution of myocardial inflammation without further relapse or sequelae. However, the disease has been observed to recur in a similar scenario to initial presentation, which then may resolve spontaneously or be associated with heart failure, arrhythmias, or death. Chronic myocarditis may be considered to be one of the mechanisms of the process of recurrence. Recurrence was reported in 10 to 25 % of patients after apparent resolution of the initial illness [58,59]. Recurrence of myocarditis is well recognized in patients with acute rheumatic fever. It is also demonstrated in subsequent pregnancies after peripartum cardiomyopathy and recurrence should be suspected if ventricular function subsequently deteriorates [59]. Women should be counseled to avoid pregnancy after a diagnosis of peripartum cardiomyopathy. Recurrence was also described in giant cell myocarditis in transplanted heart which responded to intensive immunosuppression. History of third time recurrences of active myocarditis proven by endomyocardial biopsy associated with complete atrioventricular block was described as well and viral studies showed no evidence of recent infection [60]. Another report present recurrent viral myocarditis and vaccine-associated myocarditis in a single patient with complete reversal of the cardiomyopathy and return to normal cardiac function [61]. Moreover, some cases were observed to have recurrent myocarditis after tapering of immunosuppressive therapy and previous biopsy specimens showing healed myocarditis. One report indicated that pericarditis on initial presentation may be associated with a higher rate of recurrence of myocarditis [62]. However, in reality, there are no reliable predictors that identify patients likely to have recurrence.

7. Manifestations of specific forms of myocarditis

Specific clinical forms of myocarditis of variable etiologies will be described below. Table 2 summarized some key clinical hints among specific forms of myocarditis that help with the clinical diagnosis.

7.1. Viral myocarditis

Amongst the multiple infectious etiologies which have been implicated as the cause of clinically significant acute myocarditis, viral myocarditis is the most common and the enterovirus coxsackie B the most significant. Numerous seroepidemiologic and molecular studies have linked coxsackievirus B to outbreaks of myocarditis which occurred before the 1990s. The spectrum of viruses that were detected in endomyocardial biopsy samples shifted from coxsackievirus B to adenovirus in the late 1990s. In the last decade a number of reports implicate new viruses in the etiology of myocarditis and dilated cardiomyopathy. The parvovirus B19 was identified in patients with myocarditis in Germany [63,5], and hepatitis C virus was reported in Japan [64,65] as well.

Clinical clues	Clinical diagnosis	Comments
Preceding upper respiratory febrile or flu-like illness (viral nasopharyngitis or tonsillitis)	Viral myocarditis	Often self-limited
Patients present with chronic heart failure, dilated cardiomyopathy and new arrhythmias or heart block with no response to standard care	Sarcoid myocarditis	Enlarged lymph nodes suggest systemic sarcoidosis
Cutaneous rash (pruritic, maculopapular), fever, peripheral eosinophilia or a temporal relation with recently initiated medications or the use of multiple medications	Hypersensitive/ eosinophilic myocarditis	
Patients treated with anti-neoplastic chemotherapeutic agents	Anthracyclines-induced myocarditis	
History of travel to Central or South America, Systemic or pulmonary thromboembolism	Chagas disease	The apical aneurysm is typical in advanced disease
History of residence or travel through the endemic area; previous tick bites; prior or current erythema migrans lesions and coexistence of neurologic dysfunction	Lyme disease	Varying degrees of atrioventricular conduction block is common
Previous history of rheumatic heart disease or symptoms defined by Jones criteria e.g. erythema marginatum, polyarthralgia, chorea, subcutaneous nodules fever or arthralgia	Acute rheumatic fever	
Heart failure developing in the last month of pregnancy or within 5 months following delivery	Peripartum cardiomyopathy	Higher incidence of thromboembolism (hypercoagulable state of pregnancy). More often when left ventricular ejection fraction <35 %
Sustained ventricular tachycardia in rapidly progressive heart failure associated with thymoma, autoimmune disorders, or high-grade heart block	Giant-cell myocarditis	Syncope or sudden death develop due to ventricular arrhythmias or heart block

Table 2. Some key clinical hints among specific forms of myocarditis that help with the clinical diagnosis.

Early studies suggested that cardiac involvement occurred in 3.5 to 5 % of patients during outbreaks of coxsackievirus infection [66,67]. Most cases of enteroviral myocarditis or pericarditis occur in children and young adults, two-thirds of whom males. In the majority of patients, active myocarditis remains unsuspected because the subclinical and self-limited pattern of presentation or the presence of myocarditis may be inferred only by the finding of transient electrocardiographic ST-T-wave abnormalities. In addition, subtle cardiac symptoms and signs may be overshadowed by the systemic manifestations of the underlying infection or disease process. Clinically, patients give a history of a preceding upper respiratory

http://dx.doi.org/10.5772/54362

febrile illness or a flu-like syndrome, and viral nasopharyngitis or tonsillitis may be evident. In the United States Myocarditis Treatment Trial, 89 % of subjects reported a syndrome consistent with a viral prodrome [18]. The patient may also have fever, myalgias, and muscle tenderness, that is followed by chest pain, dyspnea or arrhythmias, and occasionally heart failure. A pericardial friction rub is documented in half of cases, and the electrocardiogram shows ST-segment elevation or ST- and T-wave abnormalities. Most adults recover completely and only a minority of cases progress to chronic dilated cardiomyopathy.

In addition to the coxsackievirus B, other members of the genus Enterovirus (coxsackievirus A, echovirus, and poliovirus) and many other viruses have also been associated, less frequently, with myocarditis; these viruses include influenza virus, Epstein–Barr virus, cytomegalovirus, human herpes virus [68], and varicella-zoster virus. Myocarditis and pericarditis were reported in association with influenza virus infection during the 1918–1919 pandemic. Unusually, myocarditis has also been described as a complication of mumps in a severe but usually self-limited form. Molecular diagnostic assays have implicated mumps virus in some cases of endocardial fibroelastosis following myocarditis as well. In a recent study of 172 patients with a biopsy sample showing myocarditis, the most common viruses were parvovirus B19, 36.6 %; enterovirus, 32.6 %; co-infection with HHV-6 and parvovirus B19, 12.6 % human herpes virus 6 (HHV-6), 10.5 %; adenovirus, 8.1 % [63].

The novel influenza virus A (H1N1) pandemic began in Mexico in 2009 and rapidly spread worldwide. Cardiac complications of H1N1 infection were uncommonly reported. Sudden death as a result of myocarditis was a rare recognized complication in otherwise immunocompetent individuals, despite the absence of significant respiratory tract infection. A report from Japan described 10 patients presented with fulminant myocarditis which was confirmed by endomyocardial biopsy in 6 patients, 8 of the cases were rescued [68]. Also, influenza myocarditis was documented in a previously healthy adult due to 2009 pandemic H1N1 virus [69]. Another fatal case of acute myocarditis was reported in an immunocompetent young woman; the autopsy revealed a predominantly lymphocytic myocarditis [70]. Cases diagnosed with fulminant myocarditis were also described in pediatric population, with fatal outcomes within a 30-day of presentation [71]. Though viral myocarditis is most often self-limited and without sequelae, fulminant condition with arrhythmias, heart failure occurs. Arrhythmias are common and are occasionally difficult to manage. Patients with fulminant myocarditis may require mechanical cardiopulmonary support or cardiac transplantation, but the majority survived and many demonstrate substantial recovery of ventricular function. Patients with myocarditis and pulmonary hypertension are at a particularly high risk of death. Deaths attributed to heart failure, tachyarrhythmias, and heart block has been reported and it seems prudent to monitor the electrocardiogram of patients with arrhythmias, especially during the acute illness. In some patients, myocarditis simulates acute myocardial infarction, with chest pain, electrocardiographic changes, and elevated serum levels of myocardial enzymes. Additionally, viral myocarditis are assumed to be the major causes of chronic dilated cardiomyopathy, some cases of myocarditis may recur as well, however the number of cases with acute myocarditis that progresses to chronic dilated cardiomyopathy remains unknown.

7.2. Human immunodeficiency virus (HIV) myocarditis

The human immunodeficiency virus type I (HIV-1) infection that causes the acquired immunodeficiency syndrome (AIDS) has become a worldwide pandemic. Since its initial description 3 decades ago, a number of factors have changed, which may have altered the nature of cardiac manifestation. Notably, survival in adult with HIV infection and AIDS is now prolonged as a result of earlier detection and use of highly active antiretroviral therapy (HAART), [72,73]. At the same time, conditions such as hypertension, diabetes, hyperlipidemia, lipodystrophy and coronary artery disease appear to add further comorbidity to HIV infection [74-76]. Human immunodeficiency virus myocarditis is the most common cardiac pathologic finding at autopsy in HIV infected patients, prevalence being as high as 70 % [77,79]. Myocarditis identified at autopsy or on endomyocardial biopsy in HIV-infected patients is most often nonspecific and manifests as focal, inflammatory lymphocytic infiltrates without myocyte necrosis. However, it is uncertain whether the myocarditis so frequently observed at autopsy is clinically relevant. Myocarditis should be considered in any HIV-infected patient with dyspnea or cardiomegaly. It is present either with signs and symptoms of congestive heart failure, or asymptomatic left ventricular (LV) dysfunction at echocardiography. Of note, the clinical features of other concomitant non-cardiac disorders may mask cardiac involvement and steer to inaccurate approach, since myocardial manifestations due of HIV infection may respond at least transiently to standard therapy. A prospective long-term clinical and echocardiographic follow-up study of asymptomatic HIV-positive patients showed a mean incidence of progression to dilated cardiomyopathy of 15.9 cases per 1,000 patient/year. The precise pathogenesis of myocarditis in AIDS is unclear. Possible direct action of HIV on myocardial tissue or an autoimmune process induced by HIV, possibly in association with other cardiotropic viruses, have been proposed. It is difficult to assess the clinical significance of viral infection of the myocardium in HIV infected patients. A histologic diagnosis of myocarditis was reported in 83 % of patients with dilated cardiomyopathy. This significant proportion had focal, nonspecific lymphocytic myocarditis [80]. Dilated cardiomyopathy can be subclinical or may present with overt clinical findings. Cardiac involvement is often subclinical as echocardiographic studies have demonstrated LV dysfunction in 41 % of asymptomatic HIV-positive individuals [81]. However, in the primary care setting, AIDS cardiac complications are unusual. One autopsy series demonstrated no cardiac disease in 115 consecutive autopsies of patients who died of AIDS-related complications [79]. In one series of 416 HIV-positive patients from Rwanda without previous history of cardiovascular disease and not receiving HAART an echocardiographically evident dilated cardiomyopathy was found in 17.7 % [82]. Overt clinical involvement is seen in 10 % of HIV patients, and the most common clinically significant finding is a dilated cardiomyopathy associated with typical findings of congestive heart failure, namely edema and shortness of breath. Apart from clinical manifestations which may be a direct consequence of HIV infection, there may be consequence of possible etiologies related to non-HIV cardiotrophic viral infection, postviral autoimmune mechanism, drug toxicity, or neoplastic infiltration by Kaposi sarcoma or lymphoma.

http://dx.doi.org/10.5772/54362

Since the introduction of HAART regimens there has been a marked reduction in the incidence of myocarditis and opportunistic infections, which has led to a nearly 30 percent reduction in HIV-associated cardiomyopathy [83]. Opportunistic infections including bacteria, fungi, protozoa, and viruses are the most frequent cause of morbidity and mortality in AIDS, in 10 to 15 % of cases [84]. However, symptomatic disease appears to be rare. Toxoplasma gondii is the most frequently documented infectious cause of myocarditis associated with AIDS. Myocardial toxoplasmosis has been described in 1 to 16 % of autopsy series of patients dying of AIDS [77,78,85]. Cytomegalovirus is another common opportunistic infection in patients with late stage AIDS that can cause myocarditis [83,86]. Other virus identified within the myocardium of HIV-infected or AIDS patients, either at antemortem endomyocardial biopsy or from autopsy material, include Epstein-Barr and coxsackie B virus in adults [80,87,88]. These viruses may be present as either primary infection or as coinfection, and can occur with or without associated myocarditis and with or without associated LV dysfunction. Other infections, like myocardial tuberculosis, appears to be rare [89]. Fungal myocarditis is another unusual complication of disseminated infection that is identified most often at autopsy. Various fungal organisms have been identified in the myocardium at autopsy with associated myocarditis. Cardiac cryptococcus has been diagnosed in association with congestive heart failure and resolved after therapy [90-92].

Other possible etiologies of LV dysfunction are drug toxicity from either abuse of illicit substances, or iatrogenic disease from agents used in the therapy of AIDS. Alcohol, cocaine, or heroin may contribute to LV dysfunction in many cases [93-95]. Therapeutic agents implicated as potential cardiac toxins include zidovudine [96,97], interleukin-2 [98], and interferon alfa-2 [99,100]. Neoplastic infiltration of the heart by Kaposi sarcoma is frequently seen at autopsy and usually associated with widespread disease in the terminal phases of AIDS [101]. Non-Hodgkin lymphoma is also observed in this setting and also associated with widespread disease [102].

7.3. Bacterial myocarditis

Nowadays, myocarditis of infectious etiology caused by non-viral agents is less frequent worldwide. Bacterial involvement of the heart is uncommon, but when it does occur, it is usually as a complication of endocarditis. Various bacteria include (*Corynebacterium diphtheriae, Streptococcus pyogenes, Staphylococcus aureus, Haemophilus pneumoniae, Salmonella* spp., *Neisseria gonorrhoeae, Leptospira, Borrelia burgdorferi, Treponema pallidum, Brucella, Mycobacterium tuberculosis,* Actinomyces, *Chlamydia* spp., *Coxiella brunetti, Mycoplasma pneumoniae* and *Rickettsia* spp). Bacteria like streptococcal and staphylococcal species and *Bartonella, Brucella, Leptospira,* and *Salmonella* species can spread to the myocardium as a consequence of severe cases of endocarditis. Some forms of bacterial myocarditis will be discussed below.

7.3.1. Diphtheritic myocarditis

Worldwide, the most common bacterial cause of myocarditis is diphtheria. As early as 1806, a relationship between infection (diphtheria) and chronic heart disease was postulated, but it was not until the 1970s, with the advent of endomyocardial biopsy, that the diagnosis of myocarditis could be established during life.

The risk of developing cardiac toxicity is proportional to the severity of local infection. *Corynebacterium diphtheriae* produce toxins that inhibit protein synthesis that can cause myocarditis and lead to a dilated, flabby, hypocontractile heart. The manifestations of diphtheritic myocarditis include various arrhythmias, conduction disturbances, and dilated cardiomyopathy. Cardiomegaly and severe congestive heart failure typically appear after the first week of illness. However, clinically evident cardiac manifestations like dyspnea, muffled heart sounds, gallop rhythm or cardiac dilatation are much less common, occurring in 10 to 25 % of all patients with diphtheria [103]. Myocarditis occurred in 22 % of 656 hospitalized patients with diphtheria in the Kyrgyz Republic in 1995; 7 % of patients with myocarditis and 2 % of patients without myocarditis died [104]. Myocarditis as evidenced by electrocardiographic changes such as ST-T wave changes, QTc prolongation, and/or first-degree heart block can be detected in as many as two-thirds of cases, often occurring when local respiratory symptoms are improving [105,106]. The conduction system is frequently involved. Complete heart block from diphtheritic myocarditis was almost always fatal before temporary cardiac pacemakers were developed. Diphtheritic myocarditis is considered the most serious complication and remains the major cause of mortality [107]. The death rate is highest during the first week of illness, particularly among patients with bull-neck diphtheria and among patients with myocarditis who develop ventricular tachycardia, atrial fibrillation, or complete heart block.

7.3.2. Lyme myocarditis

Lyme disease is an inflammatory disease caused by infection with the spirochete *Borrelia burgdorferi*. In United States, carditis occurs in approximately 5 % of infected patients, while it is less frequent in Europe, affecting approximately 0.3 to 4.0 % of untreated adults [108]. This difference may be related to infection by different organisms. A careful history should address risk factors or possible evidence of *B. burgdorferi* infection particularly in the presence of atrioventricular conduction abnormalities [109]. These include history of residence or travel through an endemic area; previous tick bites; prior or current erythema migrans lesions and coexistence of neurologic dysfunction compatible with neurologic Lyme disease. Cardiac Lyme disease occurs during the early disseminated phase of the disease, usually within weeks to a few months after infection [110]. In a patient with suspected Lyme disease after a tick bite, the possibility of coinfection with Ehrlichia (ehrilichiosis) and Babesia (babesiosis) should be considered as both can also cause myocarditis.

There is a male predominance of approximately 3:1 in cardiac Lyme disease [111]. Patients with cardiac involvement may be asymptomatic and clinically unapparent. However, some patients develop symptomatic myocarditis with cardiac muscle dysfunction and/or associated pericarditis [112,113]. Symptoms mainly include palpitations, shortness of breath, chest pain, presyncope or syncope. In a review of 84 patients with Lyme carditis, the United States Centers for Disease Control and Prevention reported palpitations in 69 %, conduction abnormalities in 19 %, myocarditis in 10 % and left ventricular failure 5 % [114]. Endomyocardial biopsy samples resemble idiopathic lymphocytic myocarditis, and rarely the spirochetal organisms are identified [108,109,115]. Atrioventricular conduction block of varying degrees are the most common manifestation of Lyme carditis. In some patients, heart block is the first and only manifestation of Lyme disease [116]. Patients may present with first-degree heart block, which can progress to second-degree or complete heart block over a short period of time [117]. One review of 52 patients with Lyme carditis found that 87 % had atrioventricular block, which was usually symptomatic [109]. Wenckebach periodicity occurred in 40 % and complete atrioventricular block in 50 %; other findings include bundle branch and fascicular blocks, although rare. In another report, 38 % of patients with Lyme carditis required a temporary pacemaker [118]. Patients with a PR interval greater than 300 milliseconds carry a highest risk for progression to complete heart block, which may develop rapidly [119]. Complete heart block caused by Lyme disease typically resolves within one week, and minor conduction disturbances within six weeks [109,110]. Other reports showed heart block usually persisting for 3 to 42 days, often resolving spontaneously [108,119-121]. In Europe, scattered case reports have suggested that *B. burgdorferi* may, in isolated cases, be a cause of chronic cardiomyopathy [122,123]. This has not been shown in the United States. A small Dutch series evaluated 42 patients with dilated cardiomyopathy [112]. Nine were seropositive for anti-B. burgdorferi; six recovered fully, two had a partial response, and one showed no improvement.

7.3.3. Salmonella myocarditis

Typhoid fever is a life-threatening illness rarely complicated by myocarditis. Salmonella myocarditis may produce variable clinical manifestations from latent to severe clinical forms, such as acute congestive heart failure or sudden cardiac death [124,125]. Postmortem studies suggest that myocarditis is a major cause of sudden unexpected death in young adults and may account for 20 % of cases [16].

7.3.4. Yersinia myocarditis

Myocarditis sometimes occurs as a complication of Yersinia. Clinical evidence of Campylobacter-associated myocarditis described in association with *Campylobacter* spp. Enteritis [126]. Mild, self-limited myocarditis accompanies 10 % of cases of Yersinia-induced arthritis and can occur independently. Typical manifestations include cardiac murmurs and transient electrocardiographic abnormalities, such as prolongation of the PR interval and nonspecific ST-segment and T wave changes. The syndrome of Yersinia-induced arthritis and carditis can be confused with acute rheumatic fever.

7.3.5. Legionella myocarditis

Myocardial involvement is a rare manifestation of Legionella infection, although the most common extrapulmonary site of Legionnaires' disease is the heart. Numerous reports have described myocarditis, pericarditis, postcardiotomy syndrome, and prosthetic valve endocarditis [127-129]. Most cases have been hospital acquired. Legionella carditis in the adult population is invariably seen in association with pneumonia; however, isolated Legionella myocardial involvement without associated pneumonia has been reported [130].

7.3.6. Mycoplasma myocarditis

Cardiac abnormalities have rarely been reported in conjunction with *Mycoplasma pneumoniae* infection, including myocarditis and pericarditis [131,132]. Myocarditis has been described in rare autopsy reports as well. Cardiac manifestations include rhythm disturbances, congestive heart failure, chest pain, and conduction abnormalities on the electrocardiogram.

7.3.7. Q fever myocarditis

Myocarditis, though uncommon, may be a particularly severe manifestation of Q fever. In a study of 1070 patients with acute Q fever from southern France, 1 % had pericarditis, and 1 % had myocarditis. In other series of 1276 patients with Q fever over a 15-year period, only eight developed myocarditis but two were among the only 12 patients with Q fever who died [133]. Q fever may also cause endocarditis which usually occurs in patients with previous valvular damage or immunocompromise particularly on a bicuspid aortic valve or a prosthetic valve.

7.3.8. Chlamydial myocarditis

Chlamydial infection also has been reported in association with clinical manifestations of myocarditis [134].

7.3.9. Relapsing fever myocarditis

Relapsing fever is an arthropod-borne infection characterized by recurrent episodes of fever, caused by spirochetes of the genus Borrelia. The first episode of illness tends to be the most severe. Myocarditis appears to be common in both louse-borne and tick-borne relapsing fever. Clinical and electrocardiographic evidence of myocarditis and myocardial dysfunction includes a prolonged QTc interval, commonly a galloping third heart sound, elevated central venous pressure, arterial hypotension, and rarely pulmonary congestion. Heart involvement has been prominent in fatal cases [135].

7.4. Acute rheumatic fever

Acute rheumatic fever (ARF) is a nonsuppurative complication of group A streptococcus pharyngitis that occurs two to four weeks following infection and arises as an autoimmune response to extracellular or somatic bacterial antigens that share epitopes similar to human tissue. Rheumatic fever remains one of the most important cardiovascular diseases that cause significant cardiac morbidity and mortality in developing countries [136]. In developed countries, ARF is generally preceded by pharyngitis but not skin infection [137]. However, data from endemic regions with ARF and rheumatic heart disease suggest a less clear association [138-140]. Acute rheumatic fever occurs most frequently in children 5 to 15 years of age. The incidence of rheumatic heart disease in patients with a history of ARF is variable;

in general, valvular damage manifesting as a murmur later in life is likely to occur in about 50 % of patients with evidence of carditis at initial presentation [141,142]. The myocardial lesions consist of nonspecific lymphocytic myocarditis and Aschoff nodules. The latter are pathognomonic of ARF. Myocarditis is often indicated by cardiomegaly and/or congestive heart failure (CHF), particularly in the absence of a significant pericardial effusion. The presence of valvulitis is established clinically by auscultatory findings. Although CHF in rheumatic fever patients traditionally has been ascribed to severe myocardial inflammation, endomycardial biopsy in patients with rheumatic carditis does not show significant evidence of myocyte damage [143]. In addition, echocardiographic left ventricular ejection fraction and indices of myocardial contractility remain normal in patients with rheumatic carditis even in the presence of CHF [144]. Further, CHF occurs only in the presence of hemodynamically significant valvular lesions. The diagnosis of ARF is established largely on clinical grounds. The clinical manifestations were initially described by Jones [145]. Subsequently, guidelines for the diagnosis of rheumatic fever reviewed have been established by the American Heart Association Working Group in 2002 [146]. The five major manifestations include migratory arthritis, carditis and valvulitis, central nervous system involvement (e.g., Sydenham chorea), erythema marginatum and subcutaneous nodules. Whereas the four minor manifestations include, arthralgia, fever, elevated acute phase reactants (erythrocyte sedimentation rate, C-reactive protein) and prolonged PR interval. The probability of ARF is high in the setting of group A streptococcal infection followed by two major manifestations or one major and two minor manifestations. Strict adherence to the Jones criteria in areas of high prevalence may result in under detection of the disease. This was illustrated in a report of 555 cases of confirmed ARF among Australian aboriginals in whom monoarthritis and low-grade fever were important manifestations [147].

7.5. Chagas myocarditis

Chagas disease is a protozoan infection due to *Trypanosoma cruzi*; transmitted by an insect vector, produces an extensive myocarditis that typically becomes evident years after the initial infection. It is a major public health problem in endemic areas and in immigrants from rural Central or South America. Chagas myocarditis is by far the most common form of cardiomyopathy in Latin American countries [148]. Chagas disease consists of acute and chronic phases. During the chronic phase, many patients present the indeterminate form. The latter describes patients who have positive serology, but no symptoms, physical signs, or laboratory evidence of organ involvement [149].

7.5.1. Acute phase

The first signs of acute Chagas' disease develop at least 1 week after contact with the infected vector. Local skin indurated erythema and swelling produces the typical portal of entry lesions at the skin known as chagomas accompanied by local lymphadenopathy. The conjunctiva portal of entry may result in a unilateral painless periorbital edema and swelling of the palpebrae (Romana's sign). Infection can also occur through blood transfusion, congenital transmission, and, much less often, organ transplantation, laboratory accident, breast feeding, and oral contamination [150]. Although heart transplantation for Chagas cardiomyopathy has been successfully performed, reactivation of *Trypanosoma cruzi* is common. These initial local signs may be followed by malaise, fever sweating, myalgias anorexia; a morbilliform rash may also appear. Generalized lymphadenopathy and hepatosplenomegaly may develop. Cardiac failure occurs secondary to myocarditis; cardiac involvement is present in over 90 % of those in whom the diagnosis is made [151]. The frequency and severity of myocarditis are inversely proportional to age [152]. The acute symptoms resolve spontaneously in virtually all patients, who then enter the asymptomatic or indeterminate phase of chronic T. cruzi infection. The electrocardiogram normalizes in over 90 % of patients after one year.

The indeterminate form usually lasts 10 to 30 years and only approximately 30 % of the patients develop overt cardiac disease. Most patients remain asymptomatic throughout their life. The natural history of this phase of disease is characterized by subtle degree of cardiac involvement and gradual appearance of clinical or electrocardiographic markers of cardiac involvement, which signals the onset of the chronic phase. In one review, progression from indeterminate to the full-blown clinical form in the chronic phase occurred at approximately 2 % per year [149]. In another report, 38.3 % of patients with positive serology but without symptoms developed chagasic cardiomyopathy over a 10-year period [153]. About 50 % of patients remain with the indeterminate form indefinitely [154].

7.5.2. Chronic phase

The chronic form is characterized by dilatation of cardiac chambers, fibrosis and thinning of the ventricular wall, aneurysm formation (especially at the left ventricular apex), and mural thrombi.

Chronic progressive heart failure is the rule and is associated with poor survival. Mortality associated with the chronic phase is almost exclusively due to cardiovascular involvement. The cause of death is sudden cardiac death in 55 to 65 %, progressive heart failure in 25 to 30 %, and stroke in 10 to 15 % [155]. Symptoms and physical signs at this stage of the disease arise from three basic syndromes that often coexist in the same patient, heart failure, cardiac dysrhythmia, and thromboembolism (systemic and pulmonary). Heart failure in Chagas heart disease is usually biventricular and commonly presents with fatigue. However, right-sided failure manifested with increased jugular venous pressure, peripheral edema, ascites, and hepatomegaly is characteristically more pronounced than left-sided failure manifested with dyspnea and pulmonary rales. Both systolic and diastolic dysfunction can occur [156]. Cardiac examination typically reveals murmurs of mitral and tricuspid regurgitation, wide splitting of the second heart sound due to right bundle branch block and prominent diffuse apical thrust.

Cardiac arrhythmias may cause palpitation, lightheadedness, dizziness, or syncope. Autonomic dysfunction results in marked abnormalities in heart rate variability. Chest pain is a common symptom and usually atypical in Chagas heart disease. It may mimic angina due to abnormal coronary vasomotion postulated as underlying mechanism [157]. Sudden cardiac death accounts for 55 to 65 % of deaths in CD; the real frequency of this complication is probably underestimated, particularly in rural areas [155]. Sudden cardiac arrest can occur

http://dx.doi.org/10.5772/54362

even in previously asymptomatic patients [158]. However, most patients have severe underlying heart disease, including ventricular aneurysms at multiple sites (posterior-lateral, inferior basal, or apical), which is a characteristic finding in Chagas heart disease [158]. Sudden death is usually precipitated by exercise, and can be caused by VT or fibrillation, asystole, or complete AV block [159]. The electrocardiogram is abnormal in most patients with cardiac involvement and typically shows right bundle branch block, left anterior hemiblock and diffuse ST-T changes, which may progress to complete atrioventricular block. Ventricular arrhythmia may also be seen as premature beats that may be multiform and runs of nonsustained ventricular tachycardia. The severity of ventricular arrhythmias tends to correlate with the degree of LV dysfunction. Other changes, like abnormal Q waves, various degrees of atrioventricular block, QT interval prolongation and variation in the QT interval (QT dispersion) are frequent findings [160].Virtually all types of atrial and ventricular arrhythmias can occur; atrial fibrillation and low QRS voltage may be observed in advanced disease. A potentially serious complication of chronic Chagas heart disease is thromboembolism. In a review of 1345 autopsies, cardiac thrombus or thromboemboli were reported in 44 %; both right and left cardiac chambers being equally affected [52]. Although thromboembolic phenomena were more common in the systemic circulation, pulmonary embolism accounted for 14 % of deaths. Cardioembolism appears to be an important cause of acute ischemic stroke. One series of 94 patients with Chagas disease in Brazil reported higher rate of cardioembolism (56 versus 9 %) as compared to control group [161]. Stroke was also reported significantly more frequently in patients who had Chagas disease related cardiomyopathy compared with patients who had other cardiomyopathies (15.0 versus 6.3 %), [162]. Echocardiography or contrast ventriculography may reveal left ventricular apical aneurysm, regional wall motion abnormalities, or diffuse cardiomyopathy. The cause of death is either intractable CHF or arrhythmias, with a minority of patients dying from embolic phenomena.

7.6. Fungal myocarditis

The incidence of invasive fungal disease has dramatically increased over the past few decades corresponding to the rising number of immunocompromised patients. Cardiac fungal infection, especially myocarditis, may be difficult to recognize clinically and may in itself produce a fatal outcome. Myocardial involvement frequently occurs in disseminated fungal infection in which multiple organs are often affected. Conditions that appear predisposing to fungal infection are human immunodeficiency virus infection, medication like, corticosteroids, antineoplastic agents or broad-spectrum antibiotics, alone or in combination with invasive medical procedures [163]. Candida was the most frequently observed organism, while Aspergillus was the second most frequent fungus to involve the heart. Rarely Cryptococcus is identified as a cause of myocarditis as well.

7.7. Eosinophilic and hypersensitivity myocarditis

The association between eosinophilia (eosinophil count >500/mm3) and heart disease was first identified by Loeffler [164]. A specific eosinophilic form of myocarditis has been identified following drug-induced hypersensitivity reactions and systemic hypereosinophilic syndromes [165]. Eosinophilic myocarditis is characterized by a predominantly mature eosinophils infiltration of the myocardium and other organ systems. It occurs in association with systemic diseases such as hypereosinophilic syndrome, Churg-Strauss syndrome and Löffler's endomyocardial fibrosis. It may also occur in association with cancer, parasitic, helminthic or protozoal infections such as Chagas disease, toxoplasmosis, schistosomiasis, trichinosis, hyatid cysts and visceral larval migrans [166-168]. Eosinophilic myocarditis has been reported after vaccination for several diseases, including smallpox [169,170]. Acute eosinophilic necrotizing myocarditis is a rare aggressive form of eosinophilic myocarditis and may represent an extreme form of hypersensitivity myocarditis which is characterized by acute onset, and rapidly results in cardiovascular deterioration and circulatory collapse carrying high mortality rates [171]. The clinical manifestations of eosinophilic myocarditis may include right and left congestive heart failure, endocardial and valvular fibrosis leading to regurgitation, and formation of endocardial thrombi. Clinical awareness is warranted when presentation may mimics acute myocardial infarction, with ischemic chest pain and ST-segment elevation on electrocardiography [172]. Hypersensitivity myocarditis is a form of eosinophilic myocarditis due to autoimmune reaction affecting the heart muscle, often induced by drugs. It is often first discovered at postmortem examination. In one series, the prevalence of clinically undetected hypersensitivity myocarditis in explanted hearts ranged from 2.4 to 7 % [173]. Numerous drugs have been implicated in hypersensitivity myocarditis, including antibiotics, [174] like penicillins, cephalosporins and sulfonamides; antipsychotics, [175] like clozapine and tricyclic antidepressants [174,176,177]; other drugs like methyldopa, hydrochlorothiazide, furosemide, tetracycline, azithromycin, aminophylline, phenytoin and benzodiazepines [165,178,179]. Hypersensitivity myocarditis not always develops early in the course of medication. Patients taking the antipsychotic agent clozapine have been reported to develop myocarditis more than two years after the drug was started [180]. Prolonged continuous infusion of dobutamine has also been associated with hypersensitivity myocarditis which has been reported in 2.4 to 23 % [181,182]. Cocaine also rarely produce a hypersensitivity myocarditis, unlike the hypereosinophilic syndrome, peripheral eosinophilia is typically absent [183].

Clinically, the presentation is often heralded by fever, peripheral eosinophilia and a drug rash that occurs days to weeks after administration of a previously well-tolerated agent. Electrocardiographic abnormalities show nonspecific ST segment changes or infarct patterns [184]. Myocardial involvement varies but usually does not result in fulminant heart failure or hemodynamic collapse. However, some patients present with sudden death or rapidly progressive heart failure [172,174].

Eosinophilic myocarditis can be a manifestation of eosinophilia-myalgia syndrome, which is a multisystem disease, caused by ingestion of contaminants in L-tryptophan containing products [185], characterized by peripheral eosinophilia and generalized disabling myalgias [186]. Eosinophils, lymphocytes, macrophages, and fibroblasts accumulate in the affected tissues, but their role in pathogenesis is unclear. The disease is frequently evolves into a chronic course but can be fatal in up to 5% of patients.

http://dx.doi.org/10.5772/54362

7.8. Giant cell myocarditis

Idiopathic giant cell myocarditis is a rare inflammatory disease that often affects previously healthy young adults and is frequently a fatal type of myocarditis [187]. The pathogenesis of this disorder is not known. It is identified by the presence of multinucleated giant cells associated with eosinophils and myocyte destruction in the absence of granulomas on endomyocardial biopsy. It is thought to be primarily autoimmune in nature because of the reported comorbidity with a variety of autoimmune disorders [188], thymoma [189], and drug hypersensitivity [190]. Idiopathic giant cell myocarditis is usually a fulminant form of myocarditis, characterised by a history of rapid progression of severe heart failure associated with refractory sustained ventricular arrhythmias. Giant-cell myocarditis is sometimes distinguished from the much more common postviral myocarditis by the presence of ventricular tachycardia, heart block, and a downhill clinical course, despite optimal clinical care. In the series of 63 patients with giant cell myocarditis enrolled in the multicenter Giant Cell Myocarditis Treatment Trial, 75 % identified with heart failure symptoms as the primary presentation, 14 % with ventricular arrhythmia and heart block in 5 % [188]. Most patients will require cardiac transplantation, the median survival from the onset of symptoms is less than 6 months and has an 89 % rate of death or transplantation. This represents a significantly worse outcome compared to lymphocytic or viral myocarditis. Despite a 25 % incidence of post-transplantation recurrence of giant cell myocarditis detected by biopsy, the 5-year survival after transplantation is about 71 % which is comparable to survival after transplantation for cardiomyopathy.

7.9. Systemic lupus erythematosus myocarditis

Acute myocarditis is an uncommon manifestation of systemic lupus erythematosus (SLE), with a prevalence of 8 to 25 % in different studies [191,192]. Myocarditis is frequently asymptomatic but less often may accompany other manifestations of acute SLE. In particular, pericarditis commonly occurs in about two-thirds of patients, and generally follows a benign course; however, pericardial tamponade or constriction occur infrequently. Myocarditis generally parallels the activity of the disease and, although common histologically, rarely results in clinical heart failure unless associated with hypertension. African American ethnicity is associated with a higher risk of myocarditis compared with Hispanic and Caucasian ethnicity [191]. Myocarditis should be suspected if there is resting tachycardia disproportionate to body temperature, ST and T wave electrocardiographic abnormalities and unexplained cardiomegaly. The cardiomegaly may be associated with symptoms and signs of heart failure, conduction abnormalities or arrhythmias [193]. Patients with SLE are at increased risk for myocardial ischemia due to accelerated atherosclerosis or coronary arteritis. Endocardial involvement with fibrinous endocarditis [194] is another serious manifestation that can lead to valvular insufficiencies or embolic events. Likewise, patients with the antiphospholipid syndrome have a higher incidence of valvular disease, a variety of thrombotic disorders, myocardial infarction, pulmonary hypertension, and cardiomyopathy. Myocardial biopsy reveals mononuclear cells infiltration distinguishing active myocarditis from fibrosis and other causes of cardiomyopathy [195] or rarely cardiotoxicity induced by hydroxychloroquine [196]. Inflammation may lead to fibrosis that may be manifested clinically as dilated cardiomyopathy.

7.10. Sarcoid myocarditis

It is a granulomatous form of myocarditis. The clinical evidence of myocardial involvement is present in approximately 5 % of patients with sarcoidosis. However, an autopsy series reported higher rates of about 25 % of subclinical cardiac involvement [197-199]. The clinical manifestations of cardiac sarcoidosis are largely nonspecific and may precede, follow, or occur concurrently with involvement of other organs. Sarcoid heart disease should be considered in the evaluation of an otherwise healthy young or middle aged person with cardiac symptoms or in a patient with known sarcoidosis who develops arrhythmias, conduction disease, or heart failure. Patients who present with apparently chronic dilated cardiomyopathy yet with new ventricular arrhythmias or second-degree or third degree heart block or who do not have a response to optimal care are more likely to have cardiac sarcoidosis [20]. Cardiac symptoms were reported in 101 patients, when cardiac sarcoidosis was diagnosed in 84 % compared to 4 % in asymptomatic patients [200]. Endomyocardial biopsy shows characteristic noncaseating granulomas. However, the diagnosis can also be inferred if there is a tissue diagnosis of sarcoidosis from an extracardiac source in the presence of a cardiomyopathy of unknown origin.

Electrocardiographic abnormalities are found in nearly 70 % of patients with sarcoidosis [197]. Cardiac involvement with sarcoidosis may produce clinical symptoms and electrocardiographic findings simulating myocardial infarction. Conduction abnormalities in form of first-degree heart block due to disease of the atrioventricular node or bundle of His, and various types of intraventricular conduction defects, are common among patients with cardiac sarcoidosis [197]. These lesions may initially be silent, but can progress to complete heart block and cause syncope [201]. Sustained or nonsustained ventricular tachycardia and ventricular premature beats are the second most common presentation of cardiac sarcoidosis; electrocardiography reveals ventricular arrhythmias in as many as 22 % of patients with sarcoidosis [202]. Supraventricular arrhythmias are infrequent. Sudden death due to ventricular tachyarrhythmias or conduction block accounts for 25 to 65 % of deaths due to cardiac sarcoidosis, however, sudden death can occur in the absence of a previous cardiac event [203-205]. Both systolic and diastolic heart failure can occur. Left ventricular aneurysms develop in patients with extensive involvement of the myocardium. Mitral incompetence may occur with cardiac sarcoidosis due to associated systolic dysfunction and left ventricular dilation or due to papillary muscle involvement by sarcoid granulomas [206]. Tricuspid regurgitation with atrioventricular block secondary to infiltration of tricuspid valves and conduction system by sarcoid granulomas has been reported as well [207]. A left atrial granulomatous mass resembling myxoma has been reported too [208].

7.11. Peripartum cardiomyopathy

The syndrome is a rare disorder of pregnancy. It was recognized in 1937, as a distinct clinical entity [209]. Currently, the etiology of peripartum cardiomyopathy (PPCM) remains un-

http://dx.doi.org/10.5772/54362

clear. However, there is compelling data from animal and human studies suggesting that PPCM is actually a type of myocarditis arising from an infectious, autoimmune, or idiopathic etiology. The relationship between pregnancy and viral myocarditis was first published in 1968 [210]. Endomyocardial biopsies in women with PPCM have demonstrated myocarditis in many patients. The highest incidence of myocarditis reported in PPCM was 76 % [211], however much lower incidence was reported (8.8 %), which found to be comparable to an age and sex matched control population undergoing transplantation for idiopathic dilated cardiomyopathy (9.1 %), [212]. Viral genomes of parvovirus B19, human herpes virus 6, Epstein–Barr virus and human cytomegalovirus revealed in endomyocardial biopsy specimens from patients with PPCM [213]. Other reported data linked with Chlamydial infection [214]. Women present with heart failure during the peripartum period and become manifested in the last month of pregnancy or within 5 months of the delivery without apparent etiology for the heart failure can be found. The clinical scenario is challenging because many normal women in the last month of a normal pregnancy experience dyspnea, fatigue and ankle edema, symptoms that can mimic early congestive cardiac failure. Physical examination can be significant for signs of right and left heart failure. Symptoms and signs that should raise the suspicion of heart failure include paroxysmal nocturnal dyspnea, chest pain, nocturnal cough, new regurgitant murmurs, pulmonary rales, elevated jugular venous pressure and hepatomegaly. The electrocardiogram usually demonstrates normal sinus or sinus tachycardia rhythm, but frequent ectopy and other atrial arrhythmias may also be present. Left ventricular hypertrophy, inverted T waves, Q waves, and nonspecific ST-T changes have also been reported [215]. Recurrence in a subsequent pregnancy has been reported. However, significant improvement occurs in up to 50 % of affected women; others are left with a progressive dilated cardiomyopathy.

8. Conclusion

Myocarditis presents with a highly variable clinical scenarios. A thorough medical history with emphasis on possible causes is essential. A scrupulous awareness to ample clinical scenarios is essential for clinicians, particularly when the cases are lacking apparent etiologies, or the presentations resembles that of acute myocardial infarction, asymptomatic left ventricular systolic dysfunction, unexplained ventricular tachyarrhythmias or cardiogenic shock. Clinicians need to be attentive when evidence is present of myocardial injury not attributable to epicardial coronary artery disease, primary valvular disease or noninflammatory causes. Usually, most cases of myocarditis are self-limited and spontaneous improvement occurs in a substantial number of patients with lymphocytic disease but is rarely, if ever, observed with granulomatous myocarditis. While routine diagnostic endomyocardial biopsy is not required in most cases of suspected acute myocarditis, the need for biopsy will depend upon the time course and severity of the clinical presentation.

Better understanding of the clinicopathological that characterize the diverse clinical scenarios and more comprehensive understanding of the natural history of the various subtypes of myocarditis should assist clinicians for better approach and subsequently plan more effective therapy in the future.

Acknowledgements

The authors would like to acknowledge Sahera Khalil Al-Nnadaf (H.D) who actively contributed in preparation and assembly of this chapter.

Author details

Rafid Fayadh Al-Aqeedi

Jordanian International Hospital for Heart & Special Surgery, Cardiology & Cardiovascular Surgery Department, Erbil-Kurdistan, Iraq

References

[1] Doolan A, Langlois N, Semsarian C. Causes of sudden cardiac death in young Australians. Med J Aust 2004;180:110 -112.

[2] Fabre A, Sheppard MN. Sudden adult death syndrome and other non ischaemic causes of sudden cardiac death: a UK experience. Heart 2005;92(3):316-320.

[3] Felker GM, Hu W, Hare JM, Hruban RH, Baughman KL, Kasper EK. The spectrum of dilated cardiomyopathy: the Johns Hopkins experience with 1,278 patients. Medicine (Baltimore) 1999;78:270 –283.

[4] Brodison A, Swann JW. Myocarditis: a Review. J Infection1998, Vol.37, pp. 99-103.

[5] Mahrholdt H, Wagner A, Deluigi CC, Kispert E, Hager S, Meinhardt G. Presentation, Patterns of Myocardial Damage, and Clinical Course of Viral Myocarditis. Circulation 2006;114:1581-1590.

[6] Magnani JW, Suk-Danik HJ, Dec GW, DiSalvo TG. Survival in biopsy proven myocarditis: a long-term retrospective analysis of the histopathologic, clinical, and hemodynamic predictors. Am Heart J 2006;151(2):463-470.

[7] Aretz HT, Billingham ME, Edwards WD, Factor SM, Fallon JT, Fenoglio JJ. Myocarditis: a histopathologic definition and classification. Am J Cardiovasc Pathol 1987;1:3-14.

[8] Baughman KL. Diagnosis of myocarditis: death of Dallas criteria. Circulation 2006;113:593-595.

[9] Lieberman EB, Hutchins GM, Herskowitz A, Rose NR, Baughman KL. Clinicopathologic description of myocarditis. J Am Coll Cardiol 1991;18:1617-1626.

[10] McCarthy RE, Boehmer JP, Hruban RH, Hutchins GM, Kasper EK, Hare JM, Baughman KL. Long-term outcome of fulminant myocarditis as compared with acute (nonfulminant) myocarditis. N Engl J Med 2000;342:690-695.

[11] Kühl U, Pauschinger M, Noutsias M, Seeberg B, Bock T, Lassner D, Poller W, Kandolf R, and Schultheiss H. High prevalence of viral genomes and multiple viral infections in the myocardium of adults with "idiopathic" left ventricular dysfunction. Circulation 2005;111:887-893.

[12] Friedrich MG, Sechtem U, Schulz-Menger J, Holmvang G, Alakija P, Cooper Lt. Cardiovascular magnetic resonance in myocarditis: A JACC White Paper. J Am Coll Cardiol 2009;53:1475-1487.

[13] Caforio A, Calabrese F, Angelini A, Tona, A. Vinci, S. Bottaro, A. Ramondo, E. Carturan, S. Iliceto, G. Thiene, L. Daliento. A prospective study of biopsy-proven myocarditis: prognostic relevance of clinical and aetiopathogenetic features at diagnosis. Eur Heart J 2007;28:1326-1333.

[14] Schwartz J, Sartini D, Huber S. Myocarditis susceptibility in female mice depends upon ovarian cycle phase at infection. Virology 2004;330:16-23.

[15] Baboonian C, Treasure T. Meta-analysis of the association of enteroviruses with human heart disease. Heart 1997;78:539 –543.

[16] Feldman AM, McNamara D. Myocarditis. N Engl J Med 2000;343:1388–1398.

[17] Imazio M, Cecchi E, Demichelis B. Myopericarditis versus viral or idiopathic acute pericarditis. Heart 2008;94:498-501.

[18] Mason JW, O'Connell JB, Herskowitz A, Rose NR, McManus BM, Billingham ME, Moon TE. A clinical trial of immunosuppressive therapy for myocarditis. The Myocarditis Treatment Trial Investigators. N Engl J Med 1995;333:269–275.

[19] Ellis CR, Di Salvo T. Myocarditis: basic and clinical aspects. Cardiol Rev, Jul-Aug 2007;15(4):170-177.

[20] Yazaki Y, Isobe M, Hiramitsu S, Morimoto S, Hiroe M, Omichi C. Comparison of clinical features and prognosis of cardiac sarcoidosis and idiopathic dilated cardiomyopathy. Am J Cardiol 1998;82:537-40.

[21] Hufnagel G, Pankuweit S, Richter A, Schonian U, Maisch B. The European Study of Epidemiology and Treatment of Cardiac Inflammatory Diseases (ESETCID): first epidemiological results. Herz 2000;25:279-285.

[22] Angelini A, Calzolari V, Calabrese F, BoVa G, Maddalena F , Chioin R, Thiene G. Myocarditis mimicking acute myocardial infarction: role of endomyocardial biopsy in the differential diagnosis. Heart 2000;84:245-250.

[23] Dec GW Jr, Waldman H, Southern J, Fallon JT, Hutter AM Jr, Palacios I. Viral myocarditis mimicking acute myocardial infarction. J Am Coll Cardiol 1992;20:85-89.

[24] Sarda L, Colin P, Boccara F, Daou D, Lebtahi R, Faraggi M. Myocarditis in patients with clinical presentation of myocardial infarction and normal coronary angiograms. J Am Coll Cardiol 2001;37:786-792.

[25] McCully RB, Cooper LT, Schreiter S. Coronary artery spasm in lymphocytic myocarditis: a rare cause of acute myocardial infarction. Heart 2005;9:202.

[26] Morgera T, Di Lenarda A, Dreas L, Pinamonti B, Humar F, Bussani R, Silvestri F, Chersevani D, Camerini F. Electrocardiography of myocarditis revisited: clinical and prognostic significance of electrocardiographic changes. Am Heart J 1992;124:455–467.

[27] Chau EM, Chow WH, Chiu C. Treatment and outcome in biopsy proven fulminant myocarditis in adults. Int J Cardiol 2006;110 (3):405-406.

[28] Khabbaz Z, Grinda JM, Fabiani JN. Extracorporeal life support: an effective and non-invasive way to treat acute necrotizing eosinophilic myocarditis. J Thorac Cardiovasc Surg 2007;133(4):1122-1124.

[29] Fuse K, Kodama M, Okura Y, Ito M, Hirono S, Kato K, Hanawa H, Aizawa Y. Predictors of disease course in patients with acute myocarditis. Circulation 2000;102(23): 2829-2835.

[30] Hosenpud JD, McAnulty JH, Niles NR. Unexpected myocardial disease in patients with life threatening arrhythmias. Br Heart J 1986;56:55-61.

[31] Marboe CC, Fenoglio JJ Jr. Pathology and natural history of human myocarditis. Pathol Immunopathol Res 1988;.7:226-239.

[32] Friedman RA, Kearney DL, Moak, JP, Fenrich AL, Perry JC. Persistence of ventricular arrhythmia after resolution of occult myocarditis in children and young adults. J Am Coll Cardiol 1994;24:780-783.

[33] Strain JE, Grose RM, Factor SM, Fisher JD. Results of endomyocardial biopsy in patients with spontaneous ventricular tachycardia but without apparent structural heart disease. Circulation 1983;68:1171-1181.

[34] Sugrue DD, Holmes DR Jr, Gersh BJ, Edwards WD, McLaran CJ, Wood DL, Osborn MJ. Cardiac histologic findings in patients with life-threatening ventricular arrhythmias of unknown origin. J Am Coll Cardiol 1984;4:952-957.

[35] Vignola PA, Aonuma K, Swaye PS, Rozanski JJ, Blankstein RL, Benson J. Lymphocytic myocarditis presenting as unexplained ventricular arrhythmias: diagnosis with en-

domyocardial biopsy and response to immunosuppression. J Am Coll Cardiol 1984;4:812-819.

[36] Davidoff R, Palacios I, Southern J, Fallon JT, Newell J, Dec GW. Giant cell versus lymphocytic myocarditis. A comparison of their clinical features and long-term outcomes. Circulation 1991;83:953-961.

[37] Fleming HA, Bailey SM. Sarcoid heart disease. J R Coll Physicians Lond 1981;15:245-253.

[38] Sekiguchi M, Yazaki Y, Isobe M, Hiroe M. Cardiac sarcoidosis: diagnostic, prognostic, and therapeutic considerations. Cardiovasc Drugs Ther 1996;10:495-510.

[39] Drory Y, Turetz Y, Hiss Y, Lev B, Fisman EZ, Pines A, Kramer MR. Sudden unexpected death in persons less than 40 years of age. Am J Cardiol 1991;68:1388-1392.

[40] Eckart RE, Scoville SL, Campbell CL, Shry EA, Stajduhar KC, Potter RN, Pearse LA, Virmani R. Sudden death in young adults: a 25-year review o autopsies in military recruits. Ann Intern Med 2004;141:829-834.

[41] Maron BJ, Carney KP, Lever HM, Lewis JF, Barac I, Casey SA, Sherrid MV. Relationship of race to sudden cardiac death in competitive athletes with hypertrophic cardiomyopathy. J Am Coll Cardiol 2003;41:974-980.

[42] Theleman KP, Kuiper JJ, Roberts WC. Acute myocarditis (predominately lymphocytic) causing sudden death without heart failure. Am J Cardiol 2001;88:1078-1083.

[43] Wesslen L, Pahlson C, Lindquist O, Hjelm E, Gnarpe J, Larsson E, Baandrup U. An increase in sudden unexpected cardiac deaths among young Swedish orienteers during 1979-1992. Eur Heart J 1996;17:902-910.

[44] Maron BJ, Doerer JJ, Haas TS, Tierney DM, Mueller FO. Sudden deaths in young competitive athletes: analysis of 1866 deaths in the United States, 1980-2006. Circulation 2009;119:1085-1092.

[45] Gilbert EM, Mason JW. Immunosuppressive therapy of myocarditis. In: Engelmeier RS, JB O'Connell, eds. Drug Therapy in Dilated Cardiomyopathy and Myocarditis. New York, Marcel Dekker 1987:233-263.

[46] Bowles NE, Richardson PJ, Olsen EG, Archard LC. Detection of Coxsackie-B virus specific RNA sequences in myocardial biopsy samples from patients with myocarditis and dilated cardiomyopathy. Lancet 1986;1:1120-1128.

[47] Giacca M, Severini GM, Mestroni L, Salvi A, Lardieri G, Falaschi A, Camerini F. Low frequency of detection by nested polymerase chain reaction of enterovirus ribonucleic acid in endomyocardial tissue of patients with idiopathic dilated cardiomyopathy. J Am Coll Cardiol 1994;24:1033–1040.

[48] Martin AB, Webber S, Fricker FJ, Jaffe R, Demmler G, Kearney D, Zhang YH. Acute myocarditis: rapid diagnosis by PCR in children. Circulation 1994;90:330–339.

[49] Pauschinger M, Doerner A, Kuehl U, Schwimmbeck PL, Poller W. Enteroviral RNA replication in the myocardium of patients with left ventricular dysfunction and clinically suspected myocarditis. Circulation 1999;99:889–895.

[50] Felker GM, Thompson RE, Hare JM, Hruban RH, Clementson DE, Howard DL, Baughman KL, Kasper EK. Underlying causes and long-term survival in patients with initially unexplained cardiomyopathy. N Engl J Med 2000;342:1077-1084.

[51] Bestetti R. Stroke in a hospital-derived cohort of patients with chronic Chagas' disease. Acta Cardiol 2000;55:33-38.

[52] Samuel J, Oliveira M, Correa De Araujo RR, Navarro MA, Muccillo G. Cardiac thrombosis and thromboembolism in chronic Chagas' heart disease. Am J Cardiol 1983;52:147-151.

[53] Arteaga-Fernandez E, Barretto AC, Ianni, BM, Mady C, Lopes EA, Vianna Cd. Cardiac thrombosis and embolism in patients having died of chronic Chagas cardiopathy. Arq Bras Cardiol 1989;52:189-192.

[54] Fernandes SO, de Oliveira MS, Teixeira Vd, Almeida Hd. Endocardial thrombosis and type of left vortical lesion in chronic Chagasic patients. Arq Bras Cardiol 1987;48:17-19.

[55] Amos AM, Jaber WA, Russell SD. Improved outcomes in peripartum cardiomyopathy with contemporary. Am Heart J 2006;152:509-513.

[56] Sliwa K, Fett J, Elkayam U. Peripartum cardiomyopathy. Lancet 2006;368:687-693.

[57] Ford RF, Barton JR, O'brien JM, Hollingsworth PW . Demographics, management, and outcome of peripartum cardiomyopathy in a community hospital. Am J Obstet Gynecol 2000;182:1036-1038.

[58] Daly K, Richardson PJ, Olsen EG, Bowles NE, Cunningham L. Acute myocarditis. Role of histological and virological examination in the diagnosis and assessment of immunosuppressive treatment. Br Heart J 1984;51:30-35.

[59] Dec GW Jr, Palacios IF, Fallon JT, Aretz HT, Mills J, Lee DC, Johnson RA. Active myocarditis in the spectrum of acute dilated cardiomyopathies. Clinical features, histologic correlates, and clinical outcome. N Engl J Med 1985;312:885-890.

[60] Kanazawa H, Hata N, Yamamoto E. Recurrent myocarditis of unknown etiology. J Nippon Med Sch 2004;71(4):292-296.

[61] Makaryus AN, Revere DJ, Steinberg B. Recurrent reversible dilated cardiomyopathy secondary to viral and streptococcal pneumonia vaccine associated myocarditis. Cardiol Rev 2006;14(4):e1-4.

[62] Fowler NO, Manitsas, GT. Infectious pericarditis. Prog Cardiovasc Dis 1973;16:323-336.

[63] Kuhl U, Pauschinger M, Seeberg B, Lassner D, Noutsias M, Poller W, Schultheiss HP. Viral persistence in the myocardium is associated with progressive cardiac dysfunction. Circulation 2005;112(13):1965-1970.

[64] Matsumori A. Hepatitis C virus infection and cardiomyopathies. Circ Res 2005;96:144-147.

[65] Matsumori A, Shimada T, Chapman NM, Tracy SM, Mason JW. Myocarditis and heart failure associated with hepatitis C virus infection. J Card Fail 2006;12:293-298.

[66] Gerzen P, Granath A, Holmgren B, Zetterquist S. Acute myocarditis. A follow-up study. Br Heart J 1972;34:575-583.

[67] Grist NR, Bell, EJ. Coxsackie viruses and the heart. Am Heart J 1969;77:295-300.

[68] Ukimura A, Izumi T, Matsumori A. Clinical Research Committee on Myocarditis Associated with 2009 Influenza A (H1N1) Pandemic in Japan organized by Japanese Circulation Society. Collaborators (16) . A national survey on myocarditis associated with the 2009 influenza A (H1N1) pandemic in Japan. Circ J 2010;74(10):2193-2199.

[69] Haessler S, Paez A, Rothberg M, Higgins T. 2009 Pandemic H1N1-associated Myocarditis in a Previously Healthy Adult. Clin Microbiol Infect 2010;17(4):572-574.

[70] Gdynia G, Schnitzler P, Brunner E, Kandolf R, Blaker H, Daum E, Schnabel P, Schirmacher P, Roth W. Sudden death of an immunocompetent young adult caused by novel (swine origin) influenza A/H1N1-associated myocarditis. Virchows Arch 2011;458(3):371-376.

[71] Bratincsák A, El-Said HG, Bradley JS, Shayan K, Grossfeld PD, Cannavino CR. Fulminant myocarditis associated with pandemic H1N1 influenza A virus in children. J Am Coll Cardiol 2010;9:928-929.

[72] Hoover DR, Saah AJ, Bacellar H, Phair J, Detels R, Anderson R, Kaslow R A. Clinical manifestations of AIDS in the era of pneumocystis prophylaxis. Multicenter AIDS Cohort Study. N Engl J Med 1993;329:1922-1926.

[73] Palella FJ Jr, Delaney KM, Moorman AC, Loveless MO, Fuhrer J, Satten GA, Aschman DJ, Holmberg SD. Declining morbidity and mortality among patients with advanced human immunodeficiency virus infection. HIV Outpatient Study Investigators. N Engl J Med 1998;338:853-860.

[74] Fisher SD, Lipshultz SE. Epidemiology of cardiovascular involvement in HIV disease and AIDS. Ann N Y Acad Sci 2001;946:13.

[75] Friis-Møller N, Reiss P. DAD Study Group. Class of antiretroviral drugs and the risk of myocardial infarction. N Engl J Med 2007;356:1723-35.

[76] Tershakovec AM, Frank I, Rader D. HIV-related lipodystrophy and related factors. Atherosclerosis 2004;174:1-10.

[77] Anderson DW, Virmani R, Reilly JM, O'Leary T, Cunnion RE, Robinowitz M, Macher AM, Punja U, Villaflor ST, Parrillo JE, Roberts WC. Prevalent myocarditis at necropsy in the acquired immunodeficiency syndrome. J Am Coll Cardiol 1988;11:792-799.

[78] Baroldi G, Corallo S, Moroni M, Mutinelli MR, Lazzarin A, Antonacci CM, CristinaS, Negri C. Focal lymphocytic myocarditis in acquired immunodeficiency syndrome (AIDS): a correlative morphologic and clinical study in 26 consecutive fatal cases. J Am Coll Cardiol 1988;12:463-469.

[79] Lewis W. AIDS: cardiac findings from 115 autopsies. Prog Cardiovasc Dis1989:207-215.

[80] Barbaro G, Di Lorenzo G, Grisorio B, Barbarini G. Gruppo Italiano per lo Studio Cardiologico dei Pazienti Affetti da AIDS. Incidence of dilated cardiomyopathy and detection of HIV in myocardial cells of HIV-positive patients. N Engl J Med 1998;339:1093-1099.

[81] Corallo S, Mutinelli MR, Moroni M, Lazzarini A, Celano V, Repossini A, Baroldi G. Echocardiography detects myocardial damage in AIDS: prospective study in 102 patients. Eur Heart J 1988;9:887-892.

[82] Twagirumukiza M, Nkeramihigo E, Seminega B. Prevalence of dilated cardiomyopathy in HIV-infected African patients not receiving HAART: a multicenter, observational, prospective, cohort study in Rwanda. Curr HIV Res 2007;5:129-137.

[83] Barbaro G, Di Lorenzo G, Grisorio B, Barbarini G. Cardiac involvement in the acquired immunodeficiency syndrome: a multicenter clinical-pathological study. Gruppo Italiano per lo Studio Cardiologico dei pazienti affetti da AIDS Investigators. AIDS Res Hum Retroviruses 1998;14:1071-1077.

[84] Hofman P, Drici MD, Gibelin P, Michiels JF, Thyss A. Prevalence of toxoplasma myocarditis in patients with the acquired immunodeficiency syndrome. Br Heart J 1993;70:376-381.

[85] Matturri L, Quattrone P, Varesi C, Rossi L. Cardiac toxoplasmosis in pathology of acquired immunodeficiency syndrome. Panminerva Med 1990:32:194-196.

[86] Niedt GW, Schinella RA. Acquired immunodeficiency syndrome. Clinicopathologic study of 56 autopsies. Arch Pathol Lab Med 1985:109:727-734.

[87] Dittrich H, Chow L, Denaro F, Spector S. Human immunodeficiency virus, coxsackievirus, and cardiomyopathy. Ann Intern Med 1988;108:308-309.

[88] Herskowitz A, Wu TC, Willoughby S, et al. Myocarditis and cardiotropic viral infection associated with severe left ventricular dysfunction in late stage infection with human immunodeficiency virus. J Am Coll Cardiol 1994, 24:1025–1032.

[89] Miller-Catchpole R, Variakojis D, Anastasi J, Abrahams, C. The Chicago AIDS autopsy study: opportunistic infections, neoplasms, and findings from selected organ sys-

http://dx.doi.org/10.5772/54362

tems with a comparison to national data. Chicago Associated Pathologists. Mod Pathol 1989:2:277-294.

[90] Kinney EL, Monsuez JJ, Kitzis M, Vittecoq D. Treatment of AIDS-associated heart disease. Angiology 1989;40:970-976.

[91] Lafont A, Wolff M, Marche C, Clair B, Regnier B. Overwhelming myocarditis due to Cryptococcus neoformans in an AIDS patient. Lancet1987, Vol.2:1145-1146.

[92] Lewis W, Lipsick, J, Cammarosano C. Cryptococcal myocarditis in acquired immune deficiency syndrome. Am J Cardiol 1985;55:1239-1240.

[93] Brown J, King A, Francis CK. Cardiovascular effects of alcohol, cocaine, and acquired immune deficiency. Cardiovasc Clin 1991;21:341-376.

[94] Peng SK, French WJ, Pelikan PC. Direct cocaine cardiotoxicity demonstrated by endomyocardial biopsy. Arch Pathol Lab Med 1989:113:842-845.

[95] Soodini G, Morgan, JP. Can cocaine abuse exacerbate the cardiac toxicity of human immunodeficiency virus? Clin Cardiol 2001;24:177-181.

[96] d'Amati G., Kwan W, Lewis W. Dilated cardiomyopathy in a zidovudine-treated AIDS patient. Cardiovasc Pathol 1992;1:317-320.

[97] Herskowitz A, Willoughby SB, Baughman KL, Schulman SP, Bartlett JD. Cardiomyopathy associated with antiretroviral therapy in patients with HIV infection: a report of six cases. Ann Intern Med 1992;116:311-313.

[98] Samlowski WE, Ward JH, Craven CM, Freedman RA . Severe myocarditis following high-dose interleukin-2 administration. Arch Pathol Lab Med 1989;113:838-841.

[99] Deyton LR, Walker R, Kovacs JA, Herpin B, Parker M, Masur H, Fauci AS, Lane. Reversible cardiac dysfunction associated with interferon alfa therapy in AIDS patients with Kaposi's sarcoma. N Engl J Med 1989;321:1246-1249.

[100] Zimmerman S, Adkins D, Graham M, Petruska P, Bowers C. Irreversible, severe congestive cardiomyopathy occurring in association with interferon alpha therapy. Cancer Biother 1994;9:291-299.

[101] Silver MA, Macher AM, Reichert CM, Levens, D.L., Parrillo, J.E., Longo. Cardiac involvement by Kaposi's sarcoma in acquired immune deficiency syndrome (AIDS). Am J Cardiol 1984;53:983-985.

[102] Holladay AO, Siegel RJ, Schwartz DA. Cardiac malignant lymphoma in acquired immune deficiency syndrome. Cancer 1992;70:2203-2207.

[103] Morgan BC. Cardiac complications of diphtheria. Pediatrics 1963;32:549-557.

[104] Kadirova R, Kartoglu HU, Strebel, PM. Clinical characteristics and management of 676 hospitalized diphtheria cases, Kyrgyz Republic. J Infect Dis 2000;181(Suppl 1): 110-115.

[105] Boyer NH, Weinstein L. Diphtheritic myocarditis. N Engl J Med 1948;239:913-919.

[106] Lumio JT, Groundstroem KW, Melnick OB, Huhtala H, Rakhmanova AG. Electrocardiographic abnormalities in patients with diphtheria: a prospective study. Am J Med; 116:78-83.

[107] Kneen R, Nguyen MD, Solomon T, Van TTM, Hoa NTT, Long TB, Day NPJ, Hien TT. Clinical features and predictors of diphtheritic cardiomyopathy in Vietnamese children. Clin Infect Dis 2004;39:1591.

[108] Cox J, Krajden M. Cardiovascular manifestations of Lyme disease. Am Heart J 1991;122:1449- 1455.

[109] McAlister HF, Klementowicz PT, Andrews C, Fisher JD, Feld M, Furman S. Lyme carditis: an important cause of reversible heart block. Ann Intern Med 1989;110:339-345.

[110] Fish AE, Pride YB, Pinto DS. Lyme carditis. Infect Dis Clin North Am 2008;22:275-288.

[111] Vlay SC. Cardiac manifestations in Lyme disease, Coyle, P (Ed), Mosby-Yearbook, St Louis. 1993.

[112] Vlay SC, Dervan JP, Elias J, Kane PP, Dattwyler R. Ventricular tachycardia associated with Lyme carditis. Am Heart J 1991;121:1558-1560.

[113] Lorcerie B, Boutron MC, Portier H, Beuriat P, Ravisy J, Martin F . Pericardial manifestations of Lyme disease. Ann Med Interne (Paris) 1987;138:601-603.

[114] Ciesielski CA, Markowitz LE, Horsley R, Hightower AW, Russell H, Broome CV. Lyme disease surveillance in the United States, 1983-1986. Rev Infect Dis 1989;11(Suppl 6):1435- 1441.

[115] Stanek G, Klein J, Bittner R, Glogar, D. Isolation of Borrelia burgdorferi from the myocardium of a patient with longstanding cardiomyopathy. N Engl J Med 1990;322:249-252.

[116] Kimball SA, Janson PA, LaRaia PJ. Complete heart block as the sole presentation of Lyme disease. Arch Intern Med 1989;149:1897.

[117] Peeters AJ, Sedney MI, Telgt D, ten Wolde S, Nohlmans MK, Blaauw AA, van der Linden S, Dijkmans BA. Lyme borreliosis: a possible hidden cause of heart block of unknown origin in men with pacemakers. J Infect Dis 1991; 164(1):220–221.

[118] Goldings EA, Jericho J. Lyme disease. Clin Rheum Dis 1986;12:343-367.

[119] Steere AC, Batsford WP, Weinberg M, Alexander J, Berger, Wolfson S, Malawista SE. Lyme carditis: cardiac abnormalities of Lyme disease. Ann Intern Med 1980;93:8-16.

[120] Costello JM, Alexander ME, Greco KM, Perez-Atayde AR, Laussen PC. Lyme carditis in children: presentation, predictive factors, and clinical course. Pediatrics 2009;123:e835-841.

[121] van der Linde MR, Crijns HJ, Lie KI. Transient complete AV block in Lyme disease. Electrophysiologic observations. Chest 1989;96: 219-221.

[122] Bartůnek P, Gorican K, Mrázek V. Lyme borreliosis infection as a cause of dilated cardiomyopathy. Prague Med Rep 2006;107(2):213-226.

[123] Palecek T, Kuchynka P, Hulinska D, Schramlova J,Hrbackova H, Vitkova I, Simek S, Horak J, Louch WE, Linhart A. Presence of Borrelia burgdorferi in endomyocardial biopsies in patients with new-onset unexplained dilated cardiomyopathy. Med Microbiol Immunol 2010:199(2):139-143.

[124] Al-aqeedi RF, Kamha A, Al-aani FK. Salmonella myocarditis in a young adult patient presenting with acute pulmonary edema, rhabdomyolysis, and multi-organ failure. Journal of Cardiology 2009;54:475-479.

[125] Burt CR, Proudfoot JC, Roberts M, Horowitz RH. Fatal myocarditis secondary to Salmonella septicemia in a young adult. J Emerg Med 1990;8:295-297.

[126] Kotilainen P, Lehtopolku M, Hakanen AJ. Myopericarditis in a patient with Campylobacter enteritis: a case report and literature review. Scand J Infect Dis 2006;38(6-7): 549-552.

[127] Antonarakis ES, Wung PK, Durand DJ, Leyngold I, Meyerson DA. An atypical complication of atypical pneumonia. Am J Med 2006;119:824-827.

[128] Lowry PW, Tompkins LS. Nosocomial legionellosis: a review of pulmonary and extrapulmonary syndromes. Am J Infect Control 1993;21:21.

[129] Tompkins LS, Roessler BJ, Redd SC, Markowitz L E, Cohen M L. Legionella prosthetic-valve endocarditis. N Engl J Med 1988;318:530-535.

[130] Burke PT, Shah R, Thabolingam R, Saba S. Suspected Legionella-induced perimyocarditis in an adult in the absence of pneumonia: a rare clinical entity. Tex Heart Inst J 2009;36(6):601- 603.

[131] Martin RE, Bates, JH. Atypical pneumonia. Infect Dis Clin North Am 1991;5:585.

[132] Paz A, Potasman I. Mycoplasma-associated carditis. Case reports and review. Cardiology 2002:97(2):83-88.

[133] Fournie r PE, Etienne J, Harle JR, Habib G, Raoult D. Myocarditis, a rare but severe manifestation of Q fever: report of 8 cases and review of the literature. Clin Infect Dis 2001;32:1440-1447.

[134] Mavrogeni S, Manoussakis M, Spargias K, Kolovou G,; Saroglou G,; Cokkinos DV. Myocardial involvement in a patient with chlamydia trachomatis infection. J Card Fail 2008;14(4):351- 353.

[135] Wengrower D, Knobler H, Gillis S, Chajek-Shaul T. Myocarditis in tick-borne relapsing fever. J Infect Dis 1984:149:1033.

[136] Hutchison SJ. Acute rheumatic fever. J Infect 1998;36:249-253.

[137] Guidelines for the diagnosis of rheumatic fever. Jones Criteria, 1992 update. Special Writing Group of the Committee on Rheumatic Fever, Endocarditis, and Kawasaki Disease of the Council on Cardiovascular Disease in the Young of the American Heart Association. JAMA 1992:268:2069.

[138] McDonald M, Currie BJ, Carapetis JR. Acute rheumatic fever: a chink in the chain that links the heart to the throat? Lancet Infect Dis 2004;4:240-245.

[139] McDonald MI, Towers RJ, Andrews RM, Benger N, Currie BJ, Carapetis JR. Low rates of streptococcal pharyngitis and high rates of pyoderma in Australian aboriginal communities where acute rheumatic fever is hyperendemic. Clin Infect Dis 2006;43:683-689.

[140] Noel TP, Zabriskie J, Macpherson CN, Perrotte G. Beta-haemolytic streptococci in school children 5-15 years of age with an emphasis on rheumatic fever, in the tri-island state of Grenada. West Indian Med J 2005;54:22.

[141] Albert DA, Harel L, Karrison T. The treatment of rheumatic carditis: a review and meta- analysis. Medicine (Baltimore) 1995;74:1.

[142] Meira ZM, Goulart EM, Colosimo EA, Mota CC. Long term follow up of rheumatic fever and predictors of severe rheumatic valvar disease in Brazilian children and adolescents. Heart 2005;91:1019-1022.

[143] Narula J, Chopra P, Talwar KK, KS Reddy, RS Vasan, R Tandon, ML Bhatia, and JF Southern. Does endomyocardial biopsy aid in the diagnosis of active rheumatic carditis? Circulation 1993;88:2198-2205.

[144] Essop MR, Wisenbaugh T, Sareli P. Evidence against a myocardial factor as the cause of left ventricular dilation in active rheumatic carditis. J Am Coll Cardiol 1993;22:826-829.

[145] Jones TD. The diagnosis of rheumatic fever. JAMA 1944;126:481-484.

[146] Ferrieri P. Jones Criteria Working Group. Proceedings of the Jones Criteria workshop. Circulation 2002;106:2521-2523.

[147] Carapetis JR, Currie BJ. Rheumatic fever in a high incidence population: the importance of monoarthritis and low grade fever. Arch Dis Child 2001;85:223.

[148] Schofield CJ, Dias JC. A cost-benefit analysis of Chagas disease control. Mem Inst Oswaldo Cruz 1991;86;285-295.

[149] Dias JC. The indeterminate form of human chronic Chagas' disease A clinical epidemiological review. Rev Soc Bras Med Trop 1989;22:147-156.

[150] Benchimol Barbosa PR. The oral transmission of Chagas' disease: an acute form of infection responsible for regional outbreaks. Int J Cardiol 2006;112:132-133.

[151] Pinto AY, Valente SA, Valente Vda C. Emerging acute Chagas disease in Amazonian Brazil: case reports with serious cardiac involvement. Braz J Infect Dis 2004;8:454-460.

[152] Dias JC, Kloetzel K. The prognostic value of the electrocardiographic features of chronic Chagas' disease. Rev Inst Med Trop Sao Paulo 1968;10:158-162.

[153] Coura JR, de Abreu LL, Pereira JB, Willcox HP. Morbidity in Chagas' disease. IV. Longitudinal study of 10 years in Pains and Iguatama, Minas Gerais, Brazil. Mem Inst Oswaldo Cruz 1985;80:73-80.

[154] Marin-Neto JA, Simões MV, Maciel BC. Specific diseases: cardiomyopathies and pericardial diseases. Other cardiomyopathies. In: Evidence-Based Cardiology, 2nd ed, Yusuf, S., Cairns, JA., Camm, AJ. (Eds), BMJ Books, London, 2003;718

[155] Rassi A Jr, Rassi SG, Rassi A. Sudden death in Chagas' disease. Arq Bras Cardiol 2001;76:75- 96.

[156] Sousa AC, Marin-Neto JA, Maciel BC, Gallo Júnior L, Amorim Dde S, Barreto-Martins LE. Systolic and diastolic dysfunction in the indeterminate, digestive and chronic cardiac forms of Chagas' disease. Arq Bras Cardiol 1988;50:293.

[157] Marin-Neto JA, Marzullo P, Marcassa C, Gallo Junior L, Maciel BC. Myocardial perfusion abnormalities in chronic Chagas' disease as detected by thallium-201 scintigraphy. Am J Cardiol 1992;69:780-784.

[158] Rassi Júnior A, Gabriel Rassi A, Gabriel Rassi S. Ventricular arrhythmia in Chagas disease. Diagnostic, prognostic, and therapeutic features. Arq Bras Cardiol 1995;65:377-387.

[159] Mendoza I, Camardo J, Moleiro F, Castellanos A, Medina V, Gomes J . Sustained ventricular tachycardia in chronic chagasic myocarditis: electrophysiologic and pharmacologic characteristics. Am J Cardiol 1986;57:423-427.

[160] Salles G, Xavier S, Sousa A, Hasslocher-Moreno A, Cardosa C. Prognostic value of QT interval parameters for mortality risk stratification in Chagas' disease: results of a long-term follow-up study. Circulation 2003;108:305-312.

[161] Carod-Artal FJ, Vargas AP, Horan TA, Nunes LG. Chagasic cardiomyopathy is independently associated with ischemic stroke in Chagas disease. Stroke 2005;36:965-970.

[162] Oliveira-Filho J, Viana LC, Vieira-de-Melo RM, Faiçal F, Torrea˜o JA, Villar FA, Reis FJ. Chagas disease is an independent risk factor for stroke: baseline characteristics of a Chagas Disease cohort. Stroke 2005;36:2015-2017.

[163] Nosanchuk JD. Fungal myocarditis. Front Biosci 2002;7:1423-1438.

[164] Loeffler W. Endocarditis parietalis fibroplastica mit. Bluteosinophilie.Schweiz Med Wochenschr 1936;17:817-820.

[165] Taliercio CP, Olney BA, Lie JT. Myocarditis related to drug hypersensitivity. Mayo Clin Proc 1985;60:463-468.

[166] Corradi D, Vaglio A, Maestri R, Legname V, Leonardi G, Bartoloni G, Buzio C . Eosinophilic myocarditis in a patient with idiopathic hypereosinophilic syndrome: insights into mechanisms of myocardial cell death. Hum Pathol 2004;35:1160-1163.

[167] Corssmit EP, Trip MD, Durrer JD. Löffler's endomyocarditis in the idiopathic hypereosinophilic syndrome. Cardiology 1999;91:272-276.

[168] Spodick DH. Eosinophilic myocarditis. Mayo Clin Proc 1995;72:996.

[169] Arness MK, Eckart RE, Love SS, Atwood JE, Wells TS, Engler RJ, Collins LC, Ludwig SL. Myopericarditis following smallpox vaccination. Am J Epidemiol 2004;160:642-651.

[170] Barton M, Finkelstein Y, Opavsky M, Ito S, Ho T, Ford-Jones LE, Taylor G, Benson L, Gold R. Eosinophilic myocarditis temporally with conjugate meningococcal C and hepatitis B vaccines in children. Pediatr Infect Dis J 2008;27:831-835.

[171] Cooper LT, Zehr KJ. Biventricular assist device placement and immunosuppression as therapy for necrotizing eosinophilic myocarditis. Nat Clin Pract Cardiovasc Med 2005;2:544-548.

[172] Galiuto L, Enriquez-Sarano M, Reeder GS, Tazelaar HD, Li JT, Miller FA Jr. Eosinophilic myocarditis manifesting as myocardial infarction: early diagnosis and successful treatment. Mayo Clin Proc 1997;72:603-610.

[173] Wu L, Cooper LT, Kephart G, Gleich GJ . The Eosinophil in Cardiac Disease. In: Cooper L, ed. Myocarditis: From Bench to Bedside, Humana Press, Totowa 2002:437-453.

[174] Burke AP, Saenger J, Mullick F, Virmani R. Hypersensitivity myocarditis. Arch Pathol Lab Med 1991;115:764-769.

[175] Killian JG, Kerr K, Lawrence C, Celermajer DS. Myocarditis and cardiomyopathy associated with clozapine. Lancet 1999;354:1841-1845.

[176] Ansari A, Maron BJ, Berntson DG. Drug-induced toxic myocarditis. Tex Heart Inst J 2003;30:76-79.

[177] Kounis NG, Zavras GM, Soufras GD, Kitrou M.P. Hypersensitivity myocarditis. Ann Allergy 1989;62:71-74.

[178] Ben m'rad M, Leclerc-Mercier S, Blanche P, Franck N, Rozenberg F, Fulla Y, Guesmi M, Rollot F. Drug-induced hypersensitivity syndrome: clinical and biologic disease patterns in 24 patients. Medicine (Baltimore) 2009;88:131-140.

[179] Pursnani A, Yee H, Slater W, Sarswat N. Hypersensitivity myocarditis associated with azithromycin exposure. Ann Intern Med 2009;150:225-226.

[180] Haas SJ, Hill R, Krum H, Liew D, Tonkin A, Demos L, Stephan K, McNeil JJ. Clozapine- associated myocarditis: a review of 116 cases of suspected myocarditis associated with the use of clozapine in Australia during 1993-2003. Drug Saf 2007:30:47-57.

[181] Spear GS. Eosinophilic explant carditis with eosinophilia: ? hypersensitivity to dobutamine infusion. J Heart Lung Transplant 1995;14:755-760.

[182] Takkenberg JJ, Czer LS, Fishbein MC, Luthringer DJ, Quartel AW, Mirocha J. Eosinophilic myocarditis in patients awaiting heart transplantation. Crit Care Med 2004;32:714-721.

[183] Isner JM, Chokshi, SK. Cardiovascular complications of cocaine. Curr Probl Cardiol 1991;16:89-123.

[184] Fenoglio JJ Jr, McAllister HA Jr, Mullick FG. Drug related myocarditis. I. Hypersensitivity myocarditis. Hum Pathol 1981;12:900-907.

[185] Belongia EA, Hedberg CW, Gleich GJ, White KE, Mayeno AN, Loegefing DA, Dunnette SL, Pifie PL. An investigation of the cause of the eosinophilia-myalgia syndrome associated with tryptophan use. N Engl J Med 1990;323:357-365.

[186] Martin RW, Duffy J, Engel AG, Lie JT, Bowles CA, Moyer TP, Gleich GJ. The clinical spectrum of the eosinophilia-myalgia syndrome associated with L-tryptophan ingestion. Clinical features in 20 patients and aspects of pathophysiology. Ann Intern Med 1990;113(2):124-134.

[187] Cooper LT Jr, Hare JM, Tazelaar HD, Edwards WD. Usefulness of immunosuppression for giant cell myocarditis. Am J Cardiol 2008;102:1535-1539.

[188] Cooper LT, Jr Berry GJ, Shabetai R. Idiopathic giant-cell myocarditis—natural history and treatment. Multicenter Giant Cell Myocarditis Study Group Investigators. N Engl J Med 1997;336:1860–1866.

[189] Kilgallen CM, Jackson E, Bankoff M, Salomon RN, Surks HK. A case of giant cell myocarditis and malignant thymoma: a postmortem diagnosis by needle biopsy. Clin Cardiol 1998;21:48- 51.

[190] Daniels PR, Berry GJ, Tazelaar HD, Cooper LT. Giant cell myocarditis as a manifestation of drug hypersensitivity. Cardiovasc Pathol 2000;9:287-291.

[191] Apte M, McGwin G Jr, Vilá LM, Kaslow RA, Alarcón GS, Reveille JD. Associated factors and impact of myocarditis in patients with SLE from LUMINA, a multiethnic US cohort (LV). Rheumatology (Oxford) 2008;47:362-367.

[192] Mandell BF. Cardiovascular involvement in systemic lupus erythematosus. Semin Arthritis Rheum 1987;17:126.

[193] Moder KG, Miller TD, Tazelaar HD. Cardiac involvement in systemic lupus erythematosus. Mayo Clin Proc 1999;74:275-284.

[194] Libman E, Sacks B. A hitherto undescribed form of valvular and mural endocarditis. Arch Intern Med 1924;33:701–737.

[195] Schattner A, Liang MH. The cardiovascular burden of lupus: a complex challenge. Arch Intern Med 2003;163:1507.

[196] Keating RJ, Bhatia S, Amin S, Williams A, Sinak LJ, Edwards. WD. Hydroxychloroquine-induced cardiotoxicity in a 39- year-old woman with systemic lupus erythematosus and systolic dysfunction. J Am Soc Echocardiogr 2005;18:981.

[197] Chapelon-Abric C, de Zuttere D, Duhaut P, Veyssier P, Wechsler B, Huong DLT, Godeau P, Piette JC. Cardiac sarcoidosis: a retrospective study of 41 cases. Medicine (Baltimore) 2004;83:315-334.

[198] Kim JS, Judson MA, Donnino R, Gold M, Cooper LT Jr, Prys- towsky EN. Cardiac sarcoidosis. Am Heart J 2009;157:9-21.

[199] Thomsen TK, Eriksson T. Myocardial sarcoidosis in forensic medicine. Am J Forensic Med Pathol 1999;20:52-56.

[200] Smedema JP, Snoep G, van Kroonenburgh MP, van Geuns RJ, Dassen WR . Cardiac involvement in patients with pulmonary sarcoidosis assessed at two university medical centers in the Netherlands. Chest 2005;128:30-35.

[201] Yoshida Y, Morimoto S, Hiramitsu S, Tsuboi N, Hirayama H, Itoh T . Incidence of cardiac sarcoidosis in Japanese patients with high-degree atrioventricular block. Am Heart J 1997;134:382-386.

[202] Sekiguchi M, Numao Y, Imai M, Furuie T, Mikami R. Clinical and histopathological profile of sarcoidosis of the heart and acute idiopathic myocarditis. Concepts through a study employing endomyocardial biopsy. I. Sarcoidosis. Jpn Circ J 1980;44:249-263.

[203] Reuhl J, Schneider M, Sievert H, Lutz FU, Zieger G. Myocardial sarcoidosis as a rare cause of sudden cardiac death. Forensic Sci Int 1997;89:145-153.

[204] Soejima K, Yada, H. The work-up and management of patients with apparent or subclinical cardiac sarcoidosis: with emphasis on the associated heart rhythm abnormalities. J Cardiovasc Electrophysiol 2009;20:578-583.

[205] Yazaki Y, Isobe M, Hiroe M, Morimoto S, Hiramitsu S, Nakano T, Izumi T, Sekiguchi M . Prognostic determinants of long-term survival in Japanese patients with cardiac sarcoidosis treated with prednisone. Am J Cardiol 2001;88:1006-1010.

[206] Sato Y, Matsumoto N, Kunimasa T. Multiple involvements of cardiac sarcoidosis in both left and right ventricles and papillary muscles detected by delayedenhanced magnetic resonance imaging. Int J Cardiol 2008;130:288.

[207] Goyal SB, Aragam, JR. Cardiac sarcoidosis with primary involvement of the tricuspid valve. Cardiol Rev 2006;14:e12.

[208] Abrishami B, O'Connel C, Sharma O. Cardiac sarcoidosis with presentation of large left atrial mass. Curr Opin Pulm Med 2004;10:397-400.

[209] Gouley BA, McMillan TM, bellet S. Idiopathic myocardial degeneration associated with pregnancy and especially the puerperium. Am J Med Sci 1937;19:185-199.

[210] Farber PA, Glasgow LA. Viral myocarditis during pregnancy: encephalomyocarditis virus infection in mice. Am Heart J 1970;80:96-102.

[211] Midei MG, DeMent SH, Feldman AM, Hutchins GM, Baughman KL. Peripartum myocarditis and cardiomyopathy. Circulation 1990;81:922–928.

[212] Rizeq MN, Rickenbacher PR, Fowler MB, Billingham ME . Incidence of myocarditis in peripartum cardiomyopathy. Am J Cardiol 1994;74:474-477.

[213] Bultmann BD, Klingel K, Nabauer M, Wallwiener D, Kandolf . High prevalence of viral genomes and inflammation in peripartum cardiomyopathy. Am J Obstet Gynecol 2005;193:363-365.

[214] Cenac A, Djibo A, Chaigneau C, Velmans N, Orfila J. Are anti-Chlamydia pneumoniae antibodies prognosis indicators for peripartum cardiomyopathy? J Cardiovasc Risk 2003;10:195-199.

[215] Brown CS, Bertolet BD. Peripartum cardiomyopathy: a comprehensive review. Am J Obstet Gynecol 1998;178:409-414.

Section 2

Pathogenesis

Chapter 2

Targeting T Cells to Treat *Trypanosoma cruzi*-Induced Myocarditis

Andrea Henriques-Pons and
Marcelo P. Villa-Forte Gomes

Additional information is available at the end of the chapter

http://dx.doi.org/10.5772/55301

1. Introduction

1.1. Myocarditis

In 1995, the last World Health Organization (WHO)/International Society and Federation of Cardiology (ISFC) Task Force on the definition and classification of cardiomyopathies defined myocarditis (also named "inflammatory cardiomyopathy") as an "inflammatory disease of the myocardium associated with cardiac dysfunction" [1]. In myocarditis, the inflammatory infiltrate of the myocardium is associated with necrosis and/or degeneration of adjacent myocytes, which is not typical of – nor consistent with – myocardial ischemic damage seen with coronary artery disease [1, 2]. The clinical presentation of myocarditis is dependent upon the magnitude of myocardial inflammation, thus it may be quite variable. Clinical signs and symptoms may range from subclinical disease (which may initially be unrecognized) to new-onset acute heart failure or sudden death due to ventricular arrhythmias [3]. Moreover, the clinical course of myocarditis may be as variable as its clinical presentations: some individuals may develop acute myocarditis that resolves spontaneously within a few weeks, while others may develop symptoms of chronic heart failure due to dilated cardiomyopathy (DCM) [3]. Although many patients with hemodynamically stable heart failure may respond well to optimal medical therapy, a significant percentage of patients with DCM become medically refractory and progress to irreversible end-stage heart failure for which heart transplantation becomes the only hope of survival. Indeed, it is estimated that acute myocarditis resolves completely in approximately 50% of cases, with an additional 25% of patients having incomplete recovery (i.e.; partial normalization of cardiac function), while the remainder 25% will inexorably progress to end-stage heart failure and death [1, 4-6].

Despite its seemingly over simplistic definition, myocarditis is a disease with multiple heterogeneous etiologies, which in turn lead to a highly variable and very complex pathology. The etiologies of myocarditis can be divided into three groups: infective, immune-mediated and toxic. Infective myocarditis may be bacterial (including gram-positive cocci, gram-negative rods, gram-negative cocci, mycobacterium, mycoplasma); spirochetal (Borrelia, Leptospira); fungal (including Aspergillus, Candida, Histoplasma and Cryptococcus, among others); protozoal (including *Trypanosoma cruzi, Toxoplasma gondii, Leishmania sp*); parasitic (*Tenia solium, Echinococcus granulosus, Trichinella spiralis*); rickettsial (e.g., *Coxiella burnetii*); and viral (including adenovirus, influenza A and B, Coxsakievirus, poliovirus, HIV-1, herpes simplex, and varicella-zoster, among many others). Immune-mediated myocarditis may be due to allergens (tetanus toxoid, serum sickness, drugs such as penicillin, cephalosporins, furosemide, isoniazide, tetracycline, among many others); alloantigens (as seen in heart transplant rejection); and autoantigens such as "idiopathic" (or "virus-negative") lymphocytic and giant cell myocarditis, as well as "secondary", i.e., associated with auto-immune disorders such as systemic lupus erythematosus, vasculitides, rheumatoid arthritis, myasthenia gravis, inflammatory bowel disease. Toxic myocarditis may be due to drugs (cocaine, ethanol, lithium, cyclophosphamide, etc); heavy metals (copper, iron, lead); hormones (pheochromocytoma); as well as miscellaneous etiologies such as radiation, certain spider or snake venoms, scorpion sting, arsenic, and carbon monoxide [3].

This extraordinary multitude of ethiopathogenetic agents underscores the fact that proper and accurate diagnosis of myocarditis at the tissue and molecular level is of utmost importance because it may impact therapeutic choices as well as short- and long-term prognosis. Although management of myocarditis should ideally consist of very specific and targeted therapeutic strategies that go beyond symptomatic control of heart failure and temporary reversal of cardiac dysfunction, such therapies are not clinically available for patients with most types of myocarditis.

Myocarditis should be suspected on the basis of clinical presentation and imaging data, and objective diagnosis should be made by endomyocardial biopsy (EMBx) using established histological, immunological and immunohistochemical criteria combined with molecular biological techniques, particularly polymerase chain reaction (PCR) and nested-PCR [1, 2, 7]. Histopathological analysis is essential to reach a classification of myocarditis based on histological criteria (i.e., lymphocytic, giant cell, granulomatous, etc), while semi-quantitative assessments of the specimens with regards to myocyte necrotic damage/inflammatory activity ("grading") and to measure the extension of fibrosis and architectural changes ("staging") have also been proposed [2]. Large panels of antibodies should be performed to characterize the inflammatory cell population and the activated immunological processes. Immunohistochemistry increases the sensitivity of EMBx, while amplification methods such as PCR are capable of detecting few copy viral genomes even from an extremely small amount of tissue such as an EMBx specimen [2]. A combination of these techniques will most likely reveal the pathological nature of myocarditis and help predict which patients may respond to immunomodulatory therapies or not [8].

http://dx.doi.org/10.5772/55301

2. Pathophysiology and ciinical presentation of *Trypanosoma cruzi*-induced myocarditis

In the particular case of myocarditis induced by *Trypanosoma cruzi* infection, there is a distinct disturbance in myocardial microcirculation with both vasoconstriction at the arteriolar level and coronary vasodilation, as well as microaneurysm formation and ventricular fibrosis which ultimately lead to congestive heart failure and ventricular arrhythmias [9]. Left ventricular apical aneurysm is considered to be pathognomonic of Chagas disease, consisting of thinning of the left ventricular apex, with a clear reduction of the myocardium due to fibrosis. Mural thrombus is a frequent finding. Depending on the severity of cardiac dysfunction in infected patients, the heart may maintain its normal volume or be mildly enlarged. However, patients who die of chronic advanced or acute heart failure oftentimes have severe DCM with or without hypertrophy and intramural thrombosis in the right atrium and left ventricular apex. These patients usually have rounded hearts, venous congestion, and dilated chambers mainly on the right side [10].

In this review we will focus on the importance of the acquired immune response to the control of *T. cruzi*-induced myocarditis and discuss the possibility of targeting T cells to treat the disease.

3. *Trypanosoma cruzi* infection

In 1909, Brazilian physician Carlos Chagas, M.D., identified a hemoflagellate parasite in a child's blood, leading to the discovery of the American Trypanosomiasis, or Chagas disease (named in his honor). Dr. Chagas accomplished a unique feat in the history of medicine: not only did he identify a new disease, but he also discovered the invertebrate vector and its biological characteristics; isolated the causative agent – *Trypanosoma cruzi* (named in honor of his mentor, Dr. Oswaldo Cruz) – and described its life cycle; identified the epidemiological characteristics of the disease and its symptoms; and defined the disease's diagnostic criteria. Many years later, the disease was also found to be prevalent in many other Latin American countries. Because the chronic manifestations of Chagas disease (particularly chronic heart disease) affect patients in their most productive years of life, the disease carries a heavy social and economic burden.

The disease can be transmitted by transplacental infection or during childbirth, organ transplantation, laboratory accidents with contaminated sharp objects, blood transfusion, or ingestion of food or drink contaminated with infected vectors or their feces. During the process of natural infection in endemic areas, *T. cruzi* parasites are transmitted by the infected feces of blood-sucking reduviidae bugs, mainly *Triatoma infestans* and *Rhodnius prolixus*. These insects typically live in poorly-constructed homes with cracks and crevices on the walls and roof, and are very active at night, when they feed on human blood [11]. The bugs defecate while biting exposed areas of the skin and, despite the injection of anesthetics and inhibitors of blood clothing, the person instinctively smears the bug feces into the bite. The parasite then gains access to adjacent tissue through skin breaks or mucosal surfaces such as eyes and mouth. Infective metacyclic trypomastigote forms invade macrophages and other cell types and differentiate into proliferative amastigote forms [12]. These cytoplasmic forms differentiate into trypomastigote forms that disrupt the host cell membrane and are free to be transported by blood and infect other cells, such as cardiomyocytes.

The infection is followed by a typically benign acute-phase that lasts up to two months. In this period, high numbers of circulating parasites are observed in blood. Symptoms, when present, may include fever, headache, enlarged lymph nodes, pallor, muscle pain, difficulty in breathing, swelling and abdominal or chest pain. All patients will then enter a chronic phase, which starts with a so-called "indeterminate" asymptomatic period. Most chronic patients will remain asymptomatic throughout their lives. However, about 10% will develop digestive tract (enlargement of the esophagus and/or colon, known as "megaesophagus" and "megacolon"), neurological or mixed symptoms; and about 30% will develop Chagasic myocarditis, the most common cause of death in infected patients [13].

Twenty years ago, the number of infected people was estimated at 16-18 million, with about 100 million people at risk of contracting the disease [14]. This dire epidemiological situation has improved thanks mostly to a combined effort by many Latin American countries to control the burden of transmission through insecticide spraying and serologic screening in blood banks. Contemporary estimates indicate that approximately 10 million people are infected with *T. cruzi* worldwide, and about 25 million people are considered at risk of contracting the disease [15]. Despite the reduction in the number of infected people, the dynamic movement of human populations from and to endemic areas in Latin America, the recrudescence of vector-borne transmission, the risk for domestication of silvatic species of invertebrate hosts, and the increased importance of secondary vector species still make the infection an imposing challenge [14].

An important aspect of the infection in the current globalized world is the broader geographic distribution of infected patients. In the last decades, many cases of Chagas disease were reported in the USA, Canada, Europe and some Western Pacific countries. Most of those cases were considered "imported" because they originated from infected Latin American immigrants [16]. This changing geographical distribution highlights the increasing necessity to heighten efforts to combat the spread of the disease and to develop new strategies to treat *T. cruzi*-infected patients.

4. Pathogenesis of *Trypanosoma cruzi*-induced myocarditis

In the acute phase, many cardiomyocytes are parasitized [17]. This process typically occurs in close proximity to extensive and diffuse inflammatory foci, which consists mostly of mononuclear cells. However, opposite to what is observed in the acute-phase of the disease, parasites are much less frequently found in the heart of symptomatic chronic patients, despite the persistence of extensive mononuclear inflammatory foci. Contrary to what was previously hypothesized, chronic heart involvement in Chagas disease most likely does not rely on autoimmune mechanisms, but on parasites persistence [18]. However, the reason why most patients will not develop chronic myocarditis and heart failure is unknown to this date. It is postulated that the final outcome of the infection results from a complex and random combination of pathological characteristics, including microcirculatory derangements; micro ischemia; significant impairment of the autonomic nervous system due to ganglia cells death; deregulation of the immune system balance; progressive cardiomyocytolysis induced by parasite nests; individual genetic background; malnutrition; and comorbidities.

Experiments using murine infection and *in vitro* systems showed that the innate immune response takes over the control of the infection shortly after the contact with the parasite, with NK cells producing high levels of gamma interferon (IFN-γ), which then controls the early replication of parasites in host cells [19]. Macrophages are very important to control the infection, producing nitric oxide (NO) that limits the burden of intracellular parasites. Mast cells are also very important in this scenario and we have recently published that infected CBA mice treated with cromolyn, a mast cell stabilizer, have much greater parasitemia and IFN-γ levels, and higher mortality rates, myocarditis, and cardiac damage [20].

With regards to acquired immunity, a number of published reports support the role and importance of both CD4 and CD8 T cells in the control of the infection. Experimental approaches can be used to deplete sub populations of lymphocytes, including the use of thymectomized mice; injection of neutralizing antibodies; or the infection of *nude/nude* mice [21-23]. On the other hand, human data is based on the identification of T cell subsets in postmortem specimens, which generally shows the predominance of $CD8^+$ lymphocytes with few macrophage-like, NK or plasma cells [24]. The predominance of $CD8^+$ T cells starts in the early acute-phase of the infection and extends to the chronic phase both in experimental models and human patients. Although chronic *T. cruzi*-induced myocarditis seems to have a very complex pathology, the immune system, especially $CD8^+$ T lymphocytes, is considered a key player in this condition. Despite many efforts, it is still not clear which cytotoxic cells and molecular pathways employed by T lymphocytes may be contributing to the death of cardiomyocytes. We tested whether perforin, a major cytotoxic molecule employed by $CD8^+$ T lymphocytes, was important to the death of cardiomyocytes during the infection [25]. However, we observed that the molecule was important for myocarditis control, because in the absence of this cytotoxic pathway, cardiac cellular infiltration was much more intense, but without increased signs of damage to myocytes. In this review, in this review we will summarize some data from the literature discerning biochemical pathways that target T lymphocytes migration and their effector function in the myocardium, and the possibility of targeting these cells to treat *T. cruzi*-induced myocarditis.

5. Treatment of *T. cruzi* infected patients

During the 1960s, two new drugs proved to be effective *in vitro* and *in vivo* in the treatment of Chagas disease: nifurtimox, a nitrofuran [3-methyl-4-(5-itrofurfurilidenoamino) tetrahydro-4H-1, 4-tiazin-1,1-dioxide, Bayer 2502]; and benznidazole [N-benzyl-2-nitroimidazole acetamide, RO 7-1051]. Although these drugs have been widely used since then, therapeutic efficacy varies according to the phase of the disease (acute or chronic), duration of treatment, patient's age and geographical area of original infection [13]. The best results are obtained with recently infected patients, when cure rates of 60 to 80% can be achieved, as opposed to cure rates no greater than 10% in chronic patients, depending on the severity of cardiac dysfunction [26].

The side-effects of nifurtimox include anorexia, weight loss, insomnia, nausea, vomiting, and others. Benznidazole-associated side-effects are classified in three types: (i) hypersensitivity manifestations, such as dermatitis with cutaneous eruptions, periorbital or generalized edema, fever, lymphadenopathy, and muscular and articular pain; (ii) depression of the bone marrow, among which neutropenia, granulomatosis, and thrombocytopenic purpura: (iii) peripheral polyneuropathy, in the form of paresthesia and polyneuritis.

More recently, new progenitor cell-based therapies have been developed with good and promising results. In this therapy, total bone marrow cells are collected from individual patients and a mononuclear cell-enriched preparation is slowly injected into the left and right coronary systems. No adverse effects have been described with this procedure [27] and a few months after treatment some patients had improved cardiac function. However, it is still necessary to characterize the phenotype of the transferred cells and the mechanisms underlying such improvement in cardiac function.

The lack of effective treatments for most chronic symptomatic patients reinforces the need for new drugs and strategies for treating *T. cruzi* infected patients. This could include the development of anti-parasite drugs based on the elucidation of biochemical pathways of the parasite and/or on particular aspects of the immune response triggered by the infected host.

6. Molecular therapies

Advances in basic research that focus on interconnected molecular pathways in the immune system led to the design of more specific therapeutic strategies. Many autoimmune and inflammatory diseases can be treated using humanized or fully human-derived antibodies; fusion proteins targeting co-stimulatory molecules; or injection of competitive ligands. Neutralization of molecules involved in endothelial transmigration (CD11a/CD18, for example), T lymphocyte activation (CD80/CD86 and CD28; CD25) or function (CD2, lymphocyte function-associated antigen 3 (LFA-3) and cytotoxic T-lymphocyte antigen 4 CTLA-4) are now being used with very good results [8]. However, in the case of *T. cruzi* infection, the inflammatory response is very important to control parasite burden and to maintain the immunological equilibrium during the infection. This means that an effective treatment would have to be specific enough to silence the pathogenic components of the immune system but still allow a protective response, especially to the heart. The importance of inflammation in the control of the infection is illustrated by a number of experimental approaches that block normal T cells ontogeny/development (infected nude *nu/nu*, $RAG^{-/-}$, and thymectomized mice), endothelial transmigration (blockage of adhesion molecules such as ICAM-1 and CD11a), or function (IFN-$\gamma^{-/-}$ and perforin$^{-/-}$ mice) [28, 29, 25]. In all these models, after T lymphocyte inactivation, the infection was much more aggressive with higher mortality rates and increased blood and intracellular parasitemia. Previous results indicate that this delicate balance between an efficient or harmful inflammatory response relies on multiple aspects of the normal physiology of T lymphocytes, and these may be targeted for future therapeutic strategies.

7. T lymphocyte-based possible targets for treating *T. cruzi*-induced myocarditis

7.1. T lymphocytes senescence

Immunological senescence of memory T lymphocytes is a very interesting aspect of the immune response against pathogen-based and sterile inflammation in general, not only in *T. cruzi* induced myocarditis. Normal temporary exposure of naïve T cells to antigens in an appropriate context of activation signals leads to cellular proliferation and differentiation into effector and memory T cells. Memory T lymphocytes are generated in much smaller quantities and are retained for longer periods of time to fight against a potential subsequent exposure to the same antigen, eliciting a more rapid and effective response. However, prolonged exposure of T lymphocytes to pathogen-derived antigens or endogenous danger signals leads to the accumulation of a heterogeneous memory T cell population with unique characteristics regarding the phenotypic profile and functional activities. These memory T cells are generally regarded as $CD8^+/CD28^-$ (or $CD8^+/CD57^+$) T cells, as the loss of CD28 is counterbalanced by the expression of CD57 in this population [30]. The loss of CD28 and gain of CD57 expression on T cells during persistent immune stimulation is characteristic of humans and non-human primates but probably not of mice. Although $CD8^+/CD28^-$ T cells are seen in mice, they are not the result of chronic antigenic stimulation, do not express CD57 and represent a distinct subset of naturally occurring $CD8^+$ T cells. Amongst this population ($CD8^+/CD28^-$), there is a sub population of memory T cells that was described to be increased in severe *T. cruzi*-induced myocarditis ($CD8^+/CD27^-/CD28^-$) and this particular phenotype is expressed by cells that are at the latest stage of memory activation. This means that they are closest to memory terminal differentiation and senescence, differentiated to a point where co-stimulatory signals are no longer sufficient to induce normal memory T cell response. It seems that the phenotypic sequence of memory stages is $CD27^+/CD28^+$; $CD27^-/CD28^+$ or $CD27^+/CD28^-$; and $CD27^-/CD28^-$ for cells that are 'early', 'intermediate' and 'late' stages of memory $CD8^+$ T cells, respectively [31].

It was first shown that chronic patients with cardiac enlargement and clinical or radiological evidence of heart failure have a higher frequency (%) of late activated memory $CD8^+$ T cells ($CD27^-/CD28^-$) in blood, when compared with patients that present mild cardiac alterations [32]. Accordingly, the frequency of early activated $CD27^+/CD28^+/CD8^+$ T cells in the total memory $CD8^+$ T cell population decreases, as disease becomes more severe. The authors hypothesize that there is a gradual clonal exhaustion of this sub-population of early activated memory $CD8^+$ T cells, perhaps as a result of continuous antigenic stimulation by persistent parasites

It is still not known if there is indeed a causative relation between the increase of $CD8^+/CD27^-/CD28^-$ memory cells in chronic *T. cruzi* infected patients and the more severe clinical status of myocarditis and cardiac dysfunction. However, it is interesting to speculate that these cells could have a suppressive activity over protective $CD8^+$ T lymphocytes (Fig. 1). If this is true, the death or functional suppression of protective $CD8^+$ T lymphocytes observed in severely affected patients could be a result of late stage senescent memory T cells. A similar interaction has been described for tumor cells [33]. In this case, $CD8^+/CD27^-/CD28^-$ have a suppressive activity over the proliferation of (protective) effector T lymphocytes, and this function requires cell-to-cell contact. In fact, *T. cruzi* specific late stage memory $CD4^+/CD27^-/CD28^-$ T lymphocytes are also increased in more severely affected cardiac patients, when compared with patients with mild myocarditis, as observed in the $CD8^+$ compartment [34]. It is important to highlight that these senescent memory T cells, which can be CD8 or CD4 T cells, are distinct from $CD4^+$ T regulatory (TReg) cells that express the transcriptional factor FoxP3 [35].

Although this immunological characteristic of memory T lymphocytes senescence would probably be hard to be used as a target for treatment, these peripheral blood mononuclear cells (PBMC) markers could be used as a predictive tool for the severity of potentially developing myocarditis in chronic patients in the undetermined stage.

7.2. Chemokines and T lymphocyte migration to infected myocardium

One very important aspect of the myocarditis induced by *T. cruzi* infection is to know which chemotactic mediators are produced by the cardiac tissue and which effector cells migrate to the tissue. Ultimately, the cardiac microenvironment will determine the balance between the control of parasite growth and avoidance of inflammatory secondary damage and cardiac dysfunction. In this regard, it was shown that cardiomyocytes do not act as passive players facing the infection. Indeed, these cells become activated and secrete NO, through the activity of the induced NO synthase (iNOs) enzyme; chemokines; and pro-inflammatory cytokines [36]. These mediators destroy intracellular parasites or act on inflammatory cells in the vicinity [37]. Among these mediators, we find tumor necrosis factor (TNF), interleukin (IL)-1beta (IL-1β), and chemokines growth-related oncogene (GRO or CXCL1), monokine induced by interferon-gamma (MIG or CXCL9), macrophage inflammatory protein-2 (MIP-2), interferon-gamma-inducible protein (IP-10 or CXCL10), monocyte chemotactic protein (MCP-1 or CCL2), and regulated and normal T cell expressed and secreted (RANTES or CCL5). Moreover, inflammatory cells composing cardiac inflammatory foci also produce cytokines and chemokines, composing an environment that is rich in pleiotropic inflammatory mediators.

Chemokines are small (8-14 kDa) constitutive or inducible inflammatory cytokines, comprising four protein subfamilies (CXC or α, CC or β, C or γ, and CX3C or δ) that act through transmembrane spanning G protein-coupled receptors expressed on the surface of several leukocyte and other cells. Chemokines are mostly known by their chemotactic capacity, but they also play a role in angiogenesis; dendritic cell maturation; tumor growth and metastasis; and others.

http://dx.doi.org/10.5772/55301

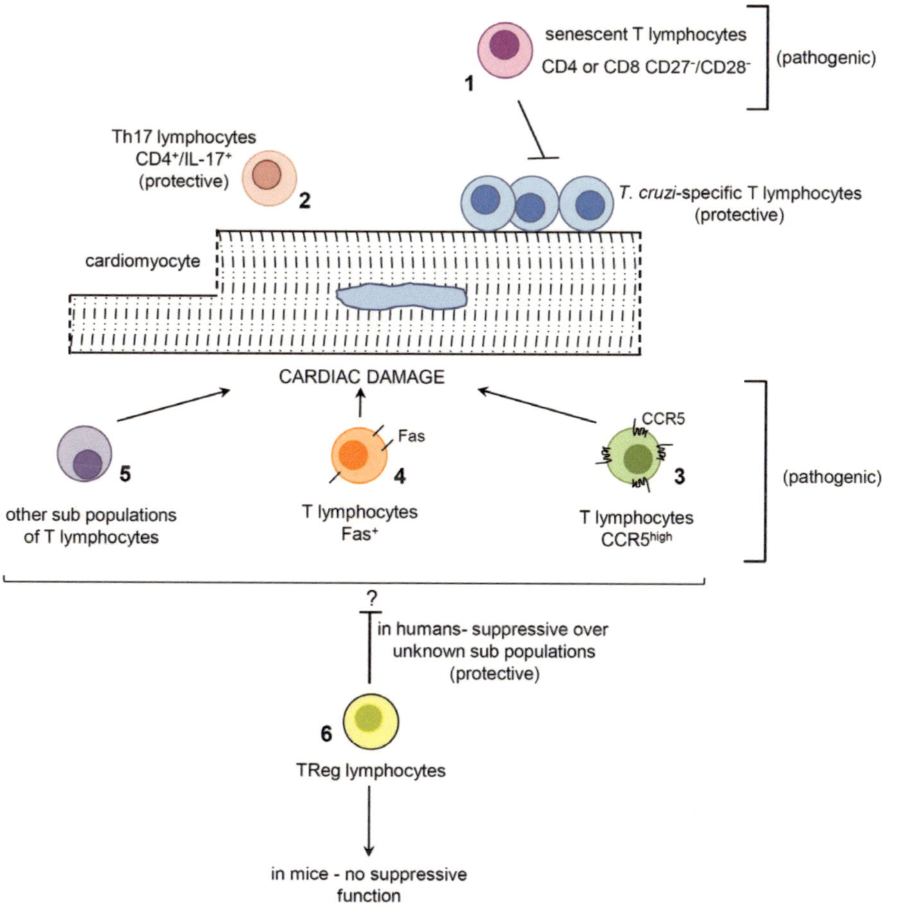

Figure 1. Cardiac pathogenic and protective T lymphocytes in *Trypanosoma cruzi* infection. Myocarditis and cardiomyocyte damage are considered pivotal in the progression of cardiac dysfunction. Therefore, the balance between pathogenic and protective T lymphocyte sub populations may determine the severity of the cardiac pathology induced by the infection. Senescent (1) CD4 and CD8 late stage memory T lymphocytes ($CD27^-/CD28^-$) are enriched in blood of patients more severely affected. It has been hypothesized that these cells act as suppressor cells over protective T lymphocytes, as observed in some tumors. $CD4^+$ T lymphocytes secreting IL-17 (Th17) (2) are protective for *T. cruzi*-induced myocarditis, as the inactivation of this cytokine leads to increased susceptibility and cardiac inflammatory infiltration. Some directly pathogenic T lymphocyte sub populations are enriched in the heart of patients with more severe myocarditis. This was observed for T lymphocytes expressing high levels of the chemokine receptor CCR5 (3), T lymphocytes (and maybe other cells, like macrophages) expressing Fas (4) and possible other pathogenic T lymphocytes that remain to be uncovered (5). T regulatory (TReg) lymphocytes apparently do not play a role in the control of myocarditis in murine infection (6), but are enriched in blood of chronic asymptomatic ones (6), when compared with cardiac symptomatic patients. Although still not known what sub populations of T lymphocytes are suppressed by TReg lymphocytes, we suggest some sub populations in the diagram. (?) Means not experimentally tested.

These functions are mostly mediated by the activation of many protein kinases, increased cytoplasmic Ca^{++} and mainly activation of transcription factors [38].

In the case of non-experimental infection with *T. cruzi*, it was found that patients with severe chronic chagasic cardiomyopathy have higher levels of TNF and CCL2 (CCR2 ligand), when compared with patients with mild cardiac dysfunction [39]. Conversely, enhanced expression of CCR5, a chemokine receptor for some CC chemokines (CCL3/MIP1α, CCL4/MIP-1β, CCL5/RANTES), and CXCR3 was found in PBMC from patients with cardiomyopathy, when compared with asymptomatic patients [40]. Taken together, these data suggest that not only cytokines, but also chemokines and their receptors, may be involved in the cardiac pathogenesis associated with *T. cruzi* infection, especially CCR5^{high} T lymphocytes (Fig. 1), what could be explored in future therapeutic designs. This is illustrated by human polymorphisms that show that migration of CCR5^{+} T lymphocytes to the heart is associated with a more severe human and experimental cardiomyopathy. Namely, studies of CCR5 59029A/G gene polymorphism in Peruvian and Venezuelan patients revealed that the G allele, which reduces CCR5 expression, is found more frequently in asymptomatic than in symptomatic chronic patients [41].

The idea that some CC chemokines, and particularly CCR5 receptor, could be involved in the pathogenesis of *T. cruzi*-induced myocarditis has been tested in experimental infection [42, 43]. Chronically infected mice were treated with N-terminal-methionylated RANTES (Met-RANTES), a selective CCR1/CCR5 antagonist, and the treatment led to a reduction in the number of cardiac parasite nests, fibrosis, and cardiomyocytes damage, as ascertained by creatine kinase (CK-MB) levels in blood. Moreover, there was an increase in the expression of connexin 43, a major component of gap junctions in the heart, and iNOs. These results are very important as a possible alternative for myocarditis treatment, especially if we consider that these mice were treated in the chronic phase, when the cardiac dysfunction is many times irreversible.

7.3. Th17 immune response

When a naïve CD4^{+} T lymphocyte encounters an antigen presenting cell (APC), it has the potential to differentiate into a T (helper) h1; Th2; Th3 (secreting mostly TGF-β and IL-10 and usually found in mucosa); inducible regulatory T lymphocyte (iTReg - cited in a following item); or Th17 lymphocyte. This commitment is mostly based on the cytokines secreted by the APC, which will interact with cognate cytokine receptors on the lymphocyte's surface and lead to the activation of the JAK/STAT (Janus kinases/Signal Transducers and Activator of Transcription proteins) pathway. The differentiation of cellular subtypes induced by the cytokines is mostly based on different combinations of JAK proteins and STAT transcription factors. In mammals, there are four members of the JAK family (JAK1, JAK2, JAK 3 and Tyk2) and seven members of the STAT family (STAT1-4; 5A; 5B; 6). These signaling molecules will ultimately induce the expression, or repression, of many genes that will orchestrate the final cellular differentiation, including the panel of cytokines that will be secreted by the final lineage committed CD4^{+} T lymphocyte [44]. Th1 cells are mainly induced by IL-12 and produce mostly IFN-γ, TNF-α, IL-2 and IL-12; while Th2 cells are mainly induced by IL-4 and produce IL4, IL5, IL-6, IL-10, and IL-13. In humans, the cytokines that instruct Th17 cell lineage development likely include IL-6; IL-21; IL-23; and IL-1β, with TGF-β playing a role in the suppression of Th1 cell lineage commitment. Then, STAT3 is necessary for gene clusters transcription, ultimately leading to the expression of their lineage-defining transcription factors, which are some retinoid orphan receptors (ROR). Th17 cells secrete mainly IL-17A, IL-17F, IL-21, IL-22, IFN-γ, IL-4, IL-10, IL-9, and IL-26 [45] and were initially described as destructive cells that induced autoimmunity and inflammatory diseases. However, more recently it became clear that they also play a role as protective cells, at least in the case of pathogenic infection with *C. albicans* and *S. aureus*.

Targeting IL-17 alone with Secukinumab (AIN457) or Ixekizumab, both fully human neutralizing antibodies against IL-17A, has been shown to lead to clinical improvement in patients with psoriasis, rheumatoid arthritis, and other auto-immune diseases. On the other hand, in the case of experimental *T. cruzi* infection, Th17 response appears to be protective against the infection (Fig. 1). IL-17A-deficient mice infected with *T. cruzi* have a lower survival rate, display prolonged and higher parasitemia, multiple organ failure, and increased markers of tissue injury when compared with infected C57BL/6 (wild type) mice [46]. Moreover, mice treated with neutralizing antibodies against IL-17 showed signs of more severe myocarditis, with more mononuclear cells migrating to the tissue [47]. According to these results, IL-17 secretion plays a role in the control of the infection and, differently from other inflammatory diseases, should not be treated by neutralizing IL-17.

7.4. Cell membrane fas/fas-L interaction

Fas agonistic stimulus was formerly a synonym of apoptosis. However, Fas/Fas-L interaction can no longer be inextricably associated with cell death. Fas-linked downstream pathways can lead to cellular survival; proliferation and/or activation, cytokines and chemokines secretion; genes transcription; inflammatory regulation; etc [8]. The Fas molecule is a type I membrane protein that belongs to the tumor necrosis factor (TNF) family, and is normally distributed as monomers on cell surface. These monomers spontaneously and temporarily group into non signaling oligomers, but agonistic activation through trimers of Fas-L leads to conformational changes and trimerization/coupling of Fas to intracellular signaling pathways. With regards to apoptosis, it has been demonstrated that two adjacent trimeric Fas complexes are sufficient to induce a functional response [48]. Alternative splicing of Fas generates soluble molecules (sFas) that retain the ability of binding to Fas-L and inhibit Fas-L-dependent responses. Fas-L is a type II membrane protein belonging to the TNF receptor family and can also exist as a membrane (mFas-L) or a soluble molecule (sFas-L). SFas-L is generated by matrix metalloproteinase (MMP7) and sFas-L monomers have no proapoptotic activity, as long as they do not induce Fas trimerization. On the other hand, sFas-L shows proinflammatory functions, acting as a strong chemotactic factor for polymorphonuclear cells, although not involved in neutrophils activation [8].

Many groups have published that Fas activation in the heart of experimental models or human patients leads to enhanced inflammation, cardiac dysfunction, and hypertrophy. Accordingly, lack of Fas/Fas-L interaction results in less severe myocarditis and cardiac involvement. To date, it has been shown that murine myocarditis induced by coxsackievirus B3 was reduced in mice treated with anti-Fas-L, in Fas-deficient mice (*lpr/lpr*), and in Fas-L-deficient mice (*gld/*

gld). In infected wild type mice, γδ T lymphocytes selectively kill protective Th2 $CD4^+$ T cells through a Fas-based pathway, enriching the inflamed heart in pathogenic Th1 cells [49]. When the Fas/Fas-L pathway is silenced, Th2 cells are enriched in the organ, what counterbalances the activity of Th1 cells and reduces cardiac inflammatory response and damage [50].

With regards to a possible molecular therapy for myocarditis that modulates Fas/Fas-L interaction, a likely alternative would involve the blockage of the pathway, which however is very complicated. The injection of competitive ligands or neutralizing Abs can mislead to general Fas inactivation and important side effects could be induced by indiscriminate lack of apoptosis, such as tumor growth and metastasis, and reduced normal turnover of cells. Moreover, the Fas/Fas-L pathway is coupled to many different cytoplasmic signaling molecules that lead to a number of different cellular responses in different populations. This makes very difficult to predict what kind of side effects could be observed [8].

In the case of myocarditis induced by *T. cruzi* infection, we observed that infected *gld/gld* mice have a very modest cardiac inflammatory infiltration, when compared with infected wild type mice, suggesting a pathogenic role for Fas-bearing cells (Fig. 1)However, despite this promising finding, we observed that both lineages have high mortality rates [51]. Apparently, the death of infected *gld/gld* mice is due to a more severe and earlier renal inflammatory infiltration/damage, while the death of infected wild type mice seems to be mostly related to myocarditis and cardiac dysfunction [52]. There are complex organ-specific modulatory roles played by Fas/Fas-L interaction, and more studies are necessary to approach this pathway therapeutically. If possible, one of the most promising options would be the injection of non-agonistic humanized Abs against Fas to avoid cardiomyocytes death through this pathway [8]. This would probably not induce bystander cell death or trigger the proinflammatory activities of this pathway. Another alternative could be the inactivation of downstream signaling molecules of the Fas pathway to reduce cardiac inflammation, hypertrophy, and dysfunction. Inhibition of Fas-1,4,5-inositol triphosphate cascade with genistein, xestospongin C, or herbimycin A prevented apoptotic and non-apoptotic cardiac dysfunction. This pathway is functionally interconnected to the PI3K/AKT/GSK3beta pathway that acts in concert to cause nuclear factor of activated T cells (NFAT) nuclear translocation. The elucidation of these Fas-based biochemical pathways responsible for unwanted outcomes in the cardiac function may help to design more efficient therapies in the future. On the other hand, it is noteworthy that any prolonged treatment blocking the Fas pathway could be dangerous.

7.5. Regulatory T cells

Regulatory T cells (TReg) were first described by Sakagushi et al [53] and consist of a thymus-derived sub-population of T lymphocytes (natural TReg cells) that have suppressive activity over effector peripheral T cells, avoiding autoimmunity. However, TReg cells can be generated in the periphery, and these cells are known as induced TReg cells. TReg cells were phenotypically described as $CD4^+/CD25^+$ and use a molecular arsenal to silence peripheral effector T cells, such as membrane IL-10 and TGF-β; CTLA-4; and others [54].

In the particular case of *T. cruzi*-induced myocarditis, there is a controversy regarding these regulatory T cells when considering animal models and results obtained from human subjects

(Fig 1). Apparently, in mice these cells have no regulatory function over effector cardiac T cells [55]. On the other hand, it was observed that these cells are enriched in chronic asymptomatic patients, when compared with chronic symptomatic ones [56]. A better discrimination of the phenotype of these cells shows that $CD4^{+}/Foxp3^{+}/CD25^{high}$ TReg cells from chronic non-cardiomyopathy patients produce higher levels of IL-17, IL-10 and granzyme B. This correlates with increased apoptosis of effector (pathogenic) cardiac T cells and maintenance of a better cardiac function [57]. Regulatory T cells would probably not be targeted for myocarditis therapy, but instead could be used as a prognostic marker for cardiac dysfunction.

8. Conclusion

All molecular pathways cited here could potentially be used to silence pathogenic T lymphocyte sub-populations that lead to myocarditis, or as a predictive tool for patients that have the potential to develop myocarditis and cardiac dysfunction. Despite this targeted modulation of sub-compartments of the immune system, the capacity of controlling the infection should in general terms be preserved to ensure infection resistance.

Author details

Andrea Henriques-Pons[1] and Marcelo P. Villa-Forte Gomes[2]

1 Laboratório de Inovações em Terapias, Ensino e Bioprodutos, Fundação Oswaldo Cruz, Instituto Oswaldo Cruz (IOC), Rio de Janeiro, Brazil

2 Cleveland Clinic, Section of Vascular Medicine, Ohio, USA

References

[1] Richardson P, McKenna W, Bristow M, Maisch B, Mautner B, O'Connell J, Olsen E, Thiene G, Goodwin J, Gyarfas I, Martin I, Nordet P: Report of the 1995 World Health Organization/International Society and Federation of Cardiology Task Force on the Definition and Classification of cardiomyopathies. Circulation 1996, 93:841-2.

[2] Basso C, Calabrese F, Angelini A, Carturan E, Thiene G: Classification and histological, immunohistochemical, and molecular diagnosis of inflammatory myocardial disease. Heart Fail Rev 2012.

[3] Caforio AL, Marcolongo R, Jahns R, Fu M, Felix SB, Iliceto S: Immune-mediated and autoimmune myocarditis: clinical presentation, diagnosis and management. Heart Fail Rev 2012.

[4] McCarthy RE, Boehmer JP, Hruban RH, Hutchins GM, Kasper EK, Hare JM, Baughman KL: Long-term outcome of fulminant myocarditis as compared with acute (nonfulminant) myocarditis. N Engl J Med 2000, 342:690-5.

[5] Kindermann I, Kindermann M, Kandolf R, Klingel K, Bültmann B, Müller T, Lindinger A, Böhm M: Predictors of outcome in patients with suspected myocarditis. Circulation 2008, 118:639-48.

[6] Jefferies JL, Towbin JA: Dilated cardiomyopathy. Lancet 2010, 375:752-62.

[7] Leone O, Veinot JP, Angelini A, Baandrup UT, Basso C, Berry G, Bruneval P, Burke M, Butany J, Calabrese F, d'Amati G, Edwards WD, Fallon JT, Fishbein MC, Gallagher PJ, Halushka MK, McManus B, Pucci A, Rodriguez ER, Saffitz JE, Sheppard MN, Steenbergen C, Stone JR, Tan C, Thiene G, van der Wal AC, Winters GL: 2011 consensus statement on endomyocardial biopsy from the Association for European Cardiovascular Pathology and the Society for Cardiovascular Pathology. Cardiovasc Pathol 2012, 21:245-74.

[8] Henriques-Pons A, de Oliveira GM: Is the Fas/Fas-L pathway a promising target for treating inflammatory heart disease? J Cardiovasc Pharmacol 2009, 53:94-9.

[9] Rossi MA, Ramos SG, Bestetti RB: Chagas' heart disease: clinical-pathological correlation. Front Biosci 2003, 8:e94-109.

[10] Higuchi MeL, Benvenuti LA, Martins Reis M, Metzger M: Pathophysiology of the heart in Chagas' disease: current status and new developments. Cardiovasc Res 2003, 60:96-107.

[11] Garcia ES, Azambuja P: Development and interactions of *Trypanosoma cruzi* within the insect vector. Parasitol Today 1991, 7:240-4.

[12] de Souza W, de Carvalho TM, Barrias ES: Review on *Trypanosoma cruzi*: Host Cell Interaction. Int J Cell Biol 2010 (doi:10.1155/2010/295394).

[13] Coura JR, Borges-Pereira J: Chagas disease. What is known and what should be improved: a systemic review. Rev Soc Bras Med Trop 2012, 45:286-96.

[14] Coura JR, Dias JC: Epidemiology, control and surveillance of Chagas disease: 100 years after its discovery. Mem Inst Oswaldo Cruz 2009, 104 Suppl 1:31-40.

[15] World Health Organization. http://www.who.int/mediacentre/factsheets/fs340/en/index.html (accessed 9 Oct 2012)

[16] Guerri-Guttenberg RA, Grana DR, Ambrosio G, Milei J: Chagas cardiomyopathy: Europe is not spared! Eur Heart J. 2008, 29(21):2587-91.

[17] Calvet CM, Melo TG, Garzoni LR, Oliveira FO, Neto DT, N S L M, Meirelles L, Pereira MC: Current understanding of the *Trypanosoma cruzi*-cardiomyocyte interaction. Front Immunol 2012, 3:327.

[18] Benvenuti LA, Roggério A, Freitas HF, Mansur AJ, Fiorelli A, Higuchi ML: Chronic American trypanosomiasis: parasite persistence in endomyocardial biopsies is associated with high-grade myocarditis. Ann Trop Med Parasitol 2008, 102:481-7.

[19] Cardillo F, Voltarelli JC, Reed SG, Silva JS: Regulation of *Trypanosoma cruzi* infection in mice by gamma interferon and interleukin 10: role of NK cells. Infect Immun 1996, 64:128-34.

[20] Meuser-Batista M, Corrêa JR, Carvalho VF, de Carvalho Britto CF, Moreira OC, Batista MM, Soares MJ, Filho FA, E Silva PM, Lannes-Vieira J, Silva RC, Henriques-Pons A: Mast cell function and death in *Trypanosoma cruzi* infection. Am J Pathol 2011, 179:1894-904.

[21] Abrahamsohn IA, Coffman RL: *Trypanosoma cruzi*: IL-10, TNF, IFN-gamma, and IL-12 regulate innate and acquired immunity to infection. Exp Parasitol 1996, 84:231-44.

[22] Da Costa SC, Calabrese KS, Bauer PG, Savino W, Lagrange PH: Studies of the thymus in Chagas' disease: III. Colonization of the thymus and other lymphoid organs of adult and newborn mice by *Trypanosoma cruzi*. Pathol Biol (Paris) 1991, 39:91-7.

[23] Russo M, Starobinas N, Minoprio P, Coutinho A, Hontebeyrie-Joskowicz M: Parasitic load increases and myocardial inflammation decreases in *Trypanosoma cruzi*-infected mice after inactivation of helper T cells. Ann Inst Pasteur Immunol 1988, 139:225-36.

[24] Reis DD, Jones EM, Tostes S, Lopes ER, Gazzinelli G, Colley DG, McCurley TL: Characterization of inflammatory infiltrates in chronic chagasic myocardial lesions: presence of tumor necrosis factor-alpha+ cells and dominance of granzyme A+, CD8+ lymphocytes. Am J Trop Med Hyg 1993, 48:637-44.

[25] Henriques-Pons A, Oliveira GM, Paiva MM, Correa AF, Batista MM, Bisaggio RC, Liu CC, Cotta-De-Almeida V, Coutinho CM, Persechini PM, Araujo-Jorge TC: Evidence for a perforin-mediated mechanism controlling cardiac inflammation in *Trypanosoma cruzi* infection. Int J Exp Pathol 2002, 83:67-79.

[26] Soeiro MN, de Castro SL: *Trypanosoma cruzi* targets for new chemotherapeutic approaches. Expert Opin Ther Targets 2009, 13:105-21.

[27] Vilas-Boas F, Feitosa GS, Soares MB, Mota A, Pinho-Filho JA, Almeida AJ, Andrade MV, Carvalho HG, Dourado-Oliveira A, Ribeiro-dos-Santos R: [Early results of bone marrow cell transplantation to the myocardium of patients with heart failure due to Chagas disease]. Arq Bras Cardiol 2006, 87:159-66.

[28] Lannes-Vieira J: *Trypanosoma cruzi*-elicited CD8+ T cell-mediated myocarditis: chemokine receptors and adhesion molecules as potential therapeutic targets to control chronic inflammation? Mem Inst Oswaldo Cruz 2003, 98:299-304.

[29] Lannes-Vieira J, Silverio JC, Pereira IR, Vinagre NF, Carvalho CM, Paiva CN, Silva da AA: Chronic *Trypanosoma cruzi*-elicited cardiomyopathy: from the discovery to

the proposal of rational therapeutic interventions targeting cell adhesion molecules and chemokine receptors--how to make a dream come true. Mem Inst Oswaldo Cruz 2009, 104 Suppl 1:226-35.

[30] Strioga M, Pasukoniene V, Characiejus D: CD8+ CD28- and CD8+ CD57+ T cells and their role in health and disease. Immunology 2011, 134:17-32.

[31] Plunkett FJ, Franzese O, Finney HM, Fletcher JM, Belaramani LL, Salmon M, Dokal I, Webster D, Lawson AD, Akbar AN: The loss of telomerase activity in highly differentiated CD8+CD28-CD27- T cells is associated with decreased Akt (Ser473) phosphorylation. J Immunol 2007, 178:7710-9.

[32] Albareda MC, Laucella SA, Alvarez MG, Armenti AH, Bertochi G, Tarleton RL, Postan M: *Trypanosoma cruzi* modulates the profile of memory CD8+ T cells in chronic Chagas' disease patients. Int Immunol 2006, 18:465-71.

[33] Montes CL, Chapoval AI, Nelson J, Orhue V, Zhang X, Schulze DH, Strome SE, Gastman BR: Tumor-induced senescent T cells with suppressor function: a potential form of tumor immune evasion. Cancer Res 2008, 68:870-9.

[34] Albareda MC, Olivera GC, Laucella SA, Alvarez MG, Fernandez ER, Lococo B, Viotti R, Tarleton RL, Postan M: Chronic human infection with *Trypanosoma cruzi* drives CD4+ T cells to immune senescence. J Immunol 2009, 183:4103-8.

[35] Wing JB, Sakaguchi S: Multiple treg suppressive modules and their adaptability. Front Immunol 2012, 3:178.

[36] Machado FS, Martins GA, Aliberti JC, Mestriner FL, Cunha FQ, Silva JS: *Trypanosoma cruzi*-infected cardiomyocytes produce chemokines and cytokines that trigger potent nitric oxide-dependent trypanocidal activity. Circulation 2000, 102:3003-8.

[37] Aliberti JC, Machado FS, Souto JT, Campanelli AP, Teixeira MM, Gazzinelli RT, Silva JS: beta-Chemokines enhance parasite uptake and promote nitric oxide-dependent microbiostatic activity in murine inflammatory macrophages infected with *Trypanosoma cruzi*. Infect Immun 1999, 67:4819-26.

[38] Blanchet X, Langer M, Weber C, Koenen RR, von Hundelshausen P: Touch of chemokines. Front Immunol 2012, 3:175.

[39] Talvani A, Rocha MO, Barcelos LS, Gomes YM, Ribeiro AL, Teixeira MM: Elevated concentrations of CCL2 and tumor necrosis factor-alpha in chagasic cardiomyopathy. Clin Infect Dis 2004, 38:943-50.

[40] Gomes JA, Bahia-Oliveira LM, Rocha MO, Busek SC, Teixeira MM, Silva JS, Correa-Oliveira R: Type 1 chemokine receptor expression in Chagas' disease correlates with morbidity in cardiac patients. Infect Immun 2005, 73:7960-6.

[41] Calzada JE, Nieto A, Beraún Y, Martín J: Chemokine receptor CCR5 polymorphisms and Chagas' disease cardiomyopathy. Tissue Antigens 2001, 58:154-8.

[42] Medeiros GA, Silvério JC, Marino AP, Roffê E, Vieira V, Kroll-Palhares K, Carvalho CE, Silva AA, Teixeira MM, Lannes-Vieira J: Treatment of chronically *Trypanosoma cruzi*-infected mice with a CCR1/CCR5 antagonist (Met-RANTES) results in amelioration of cardiac tissue damage. Microbes Infect 2009, 11:264-73.

[43] Marino AP, da Silva A, dos Santos P, Pinto LM, Gazzinelli RT, Teixeira MM, Lannes-Vieira J: Regulated on activation, normal T cell expressed and secreted (RANTES) antagonist (Met-RANTES) controls the early phase of *Trypanosoma cruzi*-elicited myocarditis. Circulation 2004, 110:1443-9.

[44] Stark GR, Darnell JE: The JAK-STAT pathway at twenty. Immunity 2012, 36:503-14.

[45] Marwaha AK, Leung NJ, McMurchy AN, Levings MK: TH17 Cells in Autoimmunity and Immunodeficiency: Protective or Pathogenic? Front Immunol 2012, 3:129.

[46] Miyazaki Y, Hamano S, Wang S, Shimanoe Y, Iwakura Y, Yoshida H: IL-17 is necessary for host protection against acute-phase *Trypanosoma cruzi* infection. J Immunol 2010, 185:1150-7.

[47] da Matta Guedes PM, Gutierrez FR, Maia FL, Milanezi CM, Silva GK, Pavanelli WR, Silva JS: IL-17 produced during *Trypanosoma cruzi* infection plays a central role in regulating parasite-induced myocarditis. PLoS Negl Trop Dis 2010, 4:e604.

[48] Holler N, Tardivel A, Kovacsovics-Bankowski M, Hertig S, Gaide O, Martinon F, Tinel A, Deperthes D, Calderara S, Schulthess T, Engel J, Schneider P, Tschopp J: Two adjacent trimeric Fas ligands are required for Fas signaling and formation of a death-inducing signaling complex. Mol Cell Biol 2003, 23(4):1428-40.

[49] Huber SA, Born W, O'Brien R: Dual functions of murine gammadelta cells in inflammation and autoimmunity in coxsackievirus B3-induced myocarditis: role of Vgamma1+ and Vgamma4+ cells. Microbes Infect 2005, 7:537-43.

[50] Seko Y, Kayagaki N, Seino K, Yagita H, Okumura K, Nagai R: Role of Fas/FasL pathway in the activation of infiltrating cells in murine acute myocarditis caused by Coxsackievirus B3. J Am Coll Cardiol 2002, 39:1399-403.

[51] de Oliveira GM, Diniz RL, Batista W, Batista MM, Bani Correa C, de Araújo-Jorge TC, Henriques-Pons A: Fas ligand-dependent inflammatory regulation in acute myocarditis induced by *Trypanosoma cruzi* infection. Am J Pathol 2007, 171:79-86.

[52] Oliveira GM, Masuda MO, Rocha NN, Schor N, Hooper CS, Araújo-Jorge TC, Henriques-Pons A: Absence of Fas-L aggravates renal injury in acute *Trypanosoma cruzi* infection. Mem Inst Oswaldo Cruz 2009, 104:1063-71.

[53] Itoh M, Takahashi T, Sakaguchi N, Kuniyasu Y, Shimizu J, Otsuka F, Sakaguchi S: Thymus and autoimmunity: production of CD25+CD4+ naturally anergic and suppressive T cells as a key function of the thymus in maintaining immunologic self-tolerance. J Immunol 1999, 162:5317-26.

[54] Schmidt A, Oberle N, Krammer PH: Molecular mechanisms of treg-mediated T cell suppression. Front Immunol 2012, 3:51.

[55] Sales PA, Golgher D, Oliveira RV, Vieira V, Arantes RM, Lannes-Vieira J, Gazzinelli RT: The regulatory CD4+CD25+ T cells have a limited role on pathogenesis of infection with *Trypanosoma cruzi*. Microbes Infect 2008, 10:680-8.

[56] de Araújo FF, Vitelli-Avelar DM, Teixeira-Carvalho A, Antas PR, Assis Silva Gomes J, Sathler-Avelar R, Otávio Costa Rocha M, Elói-Santos SM, Pinho RT, Correa-Oliveira R, Martins-Filho OA: Regulatory T cells phenotype in different clinical forms of Chagas' disease. PLoS Negl Trop Dis 2011, 5:e992.

[57] de Araújo FF, Corrêa-Oliveira R, Rocha MO, Chaves AT, Fiuza JA, Fares RC, Ferreira KS, Nunes MC, Keesen TS, Damasio MP, Teixeira-Carvalho A, Gomes JA: Foxp3+CD25(high) CD4+ regulatory T cells from indeterminate patients with Chagas disease can suppress the effector cells and cytokines and reveal altered correlations with disease severity. Immunobiology 2012, 217:768-77.

Chapter 3

Findings in Murine Viral Myocarditis

Yoshinori Seko

Additional information is available at the end of the chapter

http://dx.doi.org/10.5772/55165

1. Introduction

Acute myocarditis may not only develop into congestive heart failure, but it has also been strongly implicated in the pathogenesis of dilated cardiomyopathy. The mechanism of myocardial cell injury involved in acute myocarditis is of great clinical significance, but remained to be clarified for a long period. Because patients with acute myocarditis often show significantly increased virus titer in serum, and the myocardial histological findings of acute myocarditis are similar to those of experimental viral myocarditis, it is believed that most of human acute myocarditis is induced by virus infection. Many studies have been done on the experimental murine viral myocarditis caused by Coxsackievirus (CVB3), which is the most common pathogen of human acute myocarditis. Because maximal inflammation develops after a significant decrease in virus titer, it is thought that immunological mechanisms in addition to the direct cytolytic effects of viruses play a critical role in myocardial injury in viral myocarditis [1]. Furthermore, myocardial necrosis occurs with massive cell infiltration, strongly suggesting that cell-mediated (rather than humoral) cytotoxicity plays an important role.

Using a murine model of viral myocarditis caused by CVB3, we investigated two aspects of cell-mediated immune mechanism involved in myocardial injury. First, we analyzed the characteristics of the infiltrating immune effector cells and their mechanism of cytotoxicity, especially a role of pore-forming protein (perforin), one of the most important cytolytic effector molecules with which killer lymphocytes directly injure target cells. Second, we investigated the mechanism of infiltrating T-cell activation, usage of T-cell receptor (TCR) repertoire, expression of major histocompatibility complex (MHC) antigens, and co-stimulatory signals for T-cell activation, which are mainly mediated by members of the immunoglobulin as well as tumor necrosis factor (TNF) receptor/ligand superfamilies.

2. Characteristics of the infiltrating cells

2.1. Phenotypic analysis

There were some studies reporting the phenotypes of the immune cells playing a critical role in the development of murine viral myocarditis. These studies showed indirect evidence that T-cells, cytotoxic T-lymphocytes (CTLs), or natural killer cells (NK cells) mediated the inflammation characterized by mononuclear cell infiltration and cardiac myocyte necrosis [1-4]. However, there had been no reports directly showing the phenotypes of the infiltrating mononuclear cells and whether these infiltrating cells directly injure the cardiac myocytes. We analyzed the phenotypes of the infiltrating cells in the heart of murine viral myocarditis by immunohistochemistry with antibodies specific for NK cells, T-cells, T-helper cells (Th-cells), CTLs, and macrophages, which are the major effector cell types in cell-mediated immunity. There were almost no $\gamma\delta$ T-cells expressing TCR $\gamma\delta$. Also, we found that most of the infiltrating cells were NK cells in the early stage (on day 7 after virus infection) when maximal inflammation develops, and T-cells consisting of Th-cells and CTLs represented 10% of the infiltrating cells. The proportion of T-cells increased to 30-40% in the later stage of acute myocarditis [5]. Next, we examined the ultrastructure of the infiltrating cells by electron microscopy, and found them to be large granular lymphocytes [5]. Thus, the phenotypic and morphological analyses revealed that most of the infiltrating cells are NK-like large granular lymphocytes in the early stage when maximal inflammation develops.

2.2. Expression of a cytolytic factor perforin

NK cells and CTLs are thought to kill virus-infected cells or tumor cells by means of effector molecules contained in their cytoplasmic granules, one of which and the most important is called pore-forming protein or perforin. Perforin was shown to play a critical role in cytolysis and can be a good marker for killer lymphocytes [6-8]. To investigate whether these infiltrating cells express perforin in their cytoplasmic granules and directly injure cardiac myocytes, we examined the expression of perforin by immunohistochemistry, *in situ* hybridization, and immunoelectron microscopy. We found that about 15% of the infiltrating cells strongly expressed perforin in their cytoplasmic granules, and most of the infiltrating cells expressed perforin gene transcripts [5]. Electron microscopic analysis revealed that the infiltrating cells released massive amount of perforin molecules directly onto the surface of cardiac myocytes. There were also numerous circular lesions, consistent with pores formed by perforin on the membrane of cardiac myocytes [9]. These data clearly showed that the infiltrating cells were NK-like killer cells and directly destroy cardiac myocytes in acute myocarditis *in vivo*. We also showed the expression of perforin in the infiltrating cells in the hearts of patients with acute myocarditis and dilated cardiomyopathy [10]. These data strongly suggested that perforin-expressing killer lymphocytes play a pivotal role in myocardial inflammation. Gebhard, et al. [11] reported that perforin knockout mice infected with CVB3 develop only a mild myocarditis as compared with extensive inflammation of perforin-positive mice, whereas virus titers were indistinguishable between two groups. This supports the role of perforin in inflammation but not in virus clearance, and offers perforin to be a possible therapeutic target. However, because the strain of mice used in the study is known to develop minimal myocarditis by CVB3, further investigation using virus-sensitive strains of mice may be needed.

2.3. T–cell receptor (TCR) repertoire

Phenotypic analysis revealed that NK-like killer lymphocytes infiltrate the heart first, then infiltration by T-cells subsequently increases in the later stage. To investigate the nature of T-cell infiltration, we analyzed the expression of TCR Vβ genes in the heart of acute murine myocarditis. Polymerase chain reaction (PCR)-amplified Vβ gene products were subjected to Southern blot hybridization with a Cβ cDNA probe. We found that in contrast to spleen lymphocytes, the expression of TCR Vβ genes in the heart was restricted [12]. The restricted usage of TCR Vβ genes by infiltrating T-cells indicated that some specific antigens in the heart with viral myocarditis were being targeted. We also demonstrated the restricted usage of TCR Vα as well as Vβ genes by infiltrating cells in the hearts of patients with acute myocarditis and dilated cardiomyopathy [10]. This strongly suggested that the infiltration by T-cells recognizing some specific antigens in the heart continued, resulting in persistent myocardial cell damage, which led to the development of dilated cardiomyopathy. Because no enterovirus genomes were detected in the heart tissue by PCR in all patients, it seemed that a T-cell-mediated autoimmune mechanism may be triggered by virus infection and go on to play a pivotal role in the pathogenesis of persistent myocardial cell damage.

3. Interaction between the infiltrating cells and cardiac myocytes

3.1. Expression of major histocompatibility complex (MHC) antigens

T-cells expressing TCR αβ, consisting of CTLs and Th-cells, are known to recognize foreign antigens, such as virus-derived proteins, by their TCRs, in association with syngeneic MHC antigens on the surface of antigen-presenting cells (APCs). The recognition of MHC antigens by CTLs and Th-cells is restricted MHC classes, in general class I for CTLs and class II for Th-cells [13, 14]. To become target cells for the infiltrating T-cells, virus-infected cells need to express MHC antigens on their surfaces. To examine whether cardiac myocytes, which were reported not to express these antigens under normal conditions [15, 16], really express MHC antigens during acute viral myocarditis, we analyzed the expression of MHC antigens in hearts with acute murine myocarditis induced by CVB3. We found that CVB3-induced acute myocarditis resulted in enhanced expression of MHC class I (H-2K) antigen on cardiac myocytes adjacent to the area of cell infiltration, but undetectable or low levels of MHC class I (H-2D) or Class II (Ia) antigen were seen on cardiac myocytes, respectively [17]. The induction of MHC antigens was confirmed *in vitro* in cultured cardiac myocytes by treatment with interferon (IFN)-γ by immunohistochemistry and Northern blot analysis [17]. Induction of MHC class I antigen on cardiac myocytes with acute viral myocarditis strongly supported the interaction between cardiac myocytes and the infiltrating cells, especially CTLs, which may play a significant role in the persistent myocardial damage involved in later phase of myocarditis.

3.2. Expression of co–stimulatory molecules

It is necessary for T-cells to receive two signals from the APC for antigen-specific T-cell activation to occur. The first signal is provided by TCR engagement with the antigen-MHC complex. The second signal, that is co-stimulatory signal, is provided by co-stimulatory molecules expressed on both APC and T-cell [18]; they are mainly members of the immunoglobulin as well as TNF receptor/ligand superfamilies. A scheme showing the interaction between T-cell and APC is shown in Figure 1.

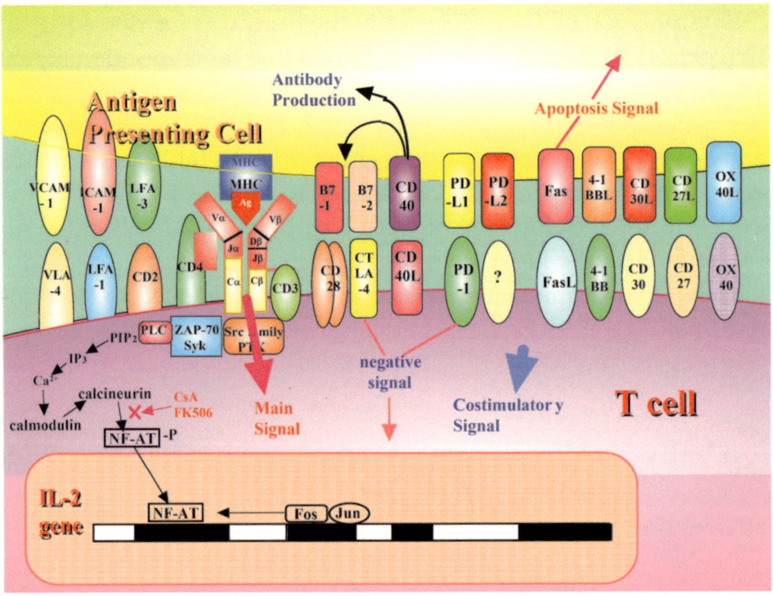

Figure 1. Interaction between T-cell and antigen-presenting cell (APC). Scheme shows pairs of receptor/ligand co-stimulatory molecules expressed on both T-cell and APC.

A. Immunoglobulin superfamily

Intercellular adhesion molecule-1 (ICAM-1]: Cell-cell interactions in the immune responses are known to be mediated by cell adhesion molecules expressed on both immune effector cells and target cells. One of the most important cell adhesion molecules is intercellular adhesion molecule-1 (ICAM-1], a ligand for lymphocyte function-associated antigen -1 (LFA-1), is expressed on most lymphocytes and thought to be induced on various target cells at the site of inflammation by cytokines [19]. ICAM-1 is known to provide a co-stimulatory signal for T-cell activation and to play an important role in the recognition, adhesion, and destruction of target cells by killer lymphocytes. Therefore, we analyzed the expression of ICAM-1 in hearts with acute murine myocarditis induced by CVB3. We found that acute myocarditis resulted in enhanced expression of ICAM-1 on cardiac myocytes, and most of the infiltrating cells expressed LFA-1 [20]. Induction of ICAM-1was also confirmed *in vitro* in cultured cardiac myocytes by treatment with IFN-γ/TNF-α by immunohistochemistry, flow cytometry, and

Northern blot analysis [20]. Because both interferon-γ and TNF-α were shown to be expressed by the infiltrating cells in the heart by *in situ* hybridization [20], the expression of ICAM-1 as well as MHC class I antigen on cardiac myocytes was thought to be induced by the infiltrating cells *in vivo*. Furthermore, we found that *In vivo* administration of an anti-ICAM-1 monoclonal antibody (mAb) significantly reduced myocardial inflammation without enhancing virus genomes in the heart [20]. We also found the expression of ICAM-1 and MHC class I antigen on cardiac myocytes and infiltration by perforin-expressing killer cells without enterovirus genomes in the heart of patients with acute myocarditis and dilated cardiomyopathy [10]. This suggested that the infiltrating killer cells may recognize some autoantigen and continuous expression of ICAM-1 as well as MHC class I antigen on cardiac myocytes may enable the infiltrating killer cells to cause persistent myocardial damage in an autoimmune phase of myocarditis, leading to dilated cardiomyopathy.

Vascular cell adhesion molecule-1 (VCAM-1): Another immunoglobulin family cell adhesion and co-stimulatory molecule, VCAM-1was also reported to be induced on myocardial cells in acute murine myocarditis. However, the role of VCAM-1 in the myocardial damage seemed to be less important than ICAM-1 [21].

B7 family molecules (B7-1, B7-2): Among the immunoglobulin superfamily co-stimulatory molecules, B7-1 and B7-2, which are the ligands for CD28 and cytotoxic T lymphocyte antigen (CTLA)-4 expressed on T-cells, have been extensively characterized and appear to be most critical [22-24]. To investigate the role of B7-1/B7-2 in the development of acute viral myocarditis, we analyzed the expression of B7-1/B7-2 in hearts with acute murine myocarditis induced by CVB3. We found that acute myocarditis strongly induced the expression of both B7-1 and B7-2 on cardiac myocytes, which normally do not express these antigens [25]. The induction of both B7-1 and B7-2 was also confirmed *in vitro* in cultured cardiac myocytes by treatment with interferon-γ. *in vivo* administration of an anti-B7-1 mAb markedly decreased myocardial inflammation, whereas an anti-B7-2 mAb-treatment abrogated the protective effect of anti-B7-1 mAb [25], indicating that different roles for B7-1 and B7-2 antigens are involved in the development of acute myocarditis. Using a murine model of chronic ongoing myocarditis, we also found that *in vivo* administration of an anti-B7-1 mAb significantly prolonged the survival of mice with myocarditis, whereas an anti-B7-2 mAb-treatment abrogated the survival-prolonging effect of anti-B7-1 mAb [26]. We found the expression of B7-1 and B7-2 on cardiac myocytes of patients with acute myocarditis and dilated cardiomyopathy [27], strongly suggesting the critical roles of these co-stimulatory molecules as in murine myocarditis. In contrast to the many co-stimulatory molecules, which deliver positive signals for T-cell activation, CTLA-4, a second B7 receptor, delivers a negative signal for T-cell activation competing with CD28. T-cell immunoglobulin mucin (Tim)-3 is highly expressed on Th1 cells, and is known to negatively regulate Th1 responses and affects susceptibility to allergy and autoimmune diseases. Frisanhco-Kiss et al. [28] reported that *in vivo* anti-Tim-3 blocking mAb-treatment reduced CTLA-4 levels in Th-cells in the spleen, and significantly increased myocardial inflammation of mice infected with CVB3. This indicates the negative regulatory role of CTLA-4 through Tim-3 signaling in viral myocarditis. Furthermore, Love et al. [29]

showed a negative regulatory role of CTLA-4 in CTLs, using a murine model of myocarditis caused by adoptive transferred antigen-specific CTLs.

Programmed death-1 (PD-1)/PD-1 ligands (PD-L1, PD-L2): Among other known co-stimulatory molecules, which mediate negative signals for T-cell activation, PD-1/PD-1 ligands, belonging to the immunoglobulin superfamily, pathway seems to be the most important [30-33]. To investigate roles of PD-1/PD-1 ligands pathway in the development of myocardial damage in murine acute myocarditis, we examined the expression of PD-L1 and PD-L2 in hearts with acute myocarditis induced by CVB3. We found that the expression of PD-L1 (but not PD-L2) was markedly induced on cardiac myocytes with acute myocarditis. The induction of PD-L1 (but not PD-L2) was also confirmed *in vitro* in cultured cardiac myocytes by treatment with IFN -γ [34]. Furthermore, *in vivo* treatment with anti-PD-1 blocking mAb significantly increased the myocardial inflammation, whereas anti-PD-1 stimulating mAb-treatment significantly decreased the myocardial inflammation. *In vivo* treatment with anti- PD-L1 blocking mAb increased the inflammation (but statistically not significant), whereas anti-PD-L2 blocking mAb-treatment had no effect [34]. This indicated that PD-1/PD-L1 pathway plays a critical role in suppressing myocardial inflammation induced by CVB3 infection.

B. TNF receptor/ligand superfamilies

Fas and Fas ligand (FasL): Fas and its ligand FasL, which belong to the TNF receptor/ligand superfamily, are well-characterized co-stimulatory molecules and known to play an essential role in the induction of apoptosis [35-38]. They are also known to play an important role in the cytotoxicity by T-cells and NK cells [39-41]. Because the percentage of cardiac myocytes undergoing apoptosis was too low to explain the mechanism involved in massive myocardial injury in acute murine myocarditis, we investigated the role of Fas/FasL pathway in the activation of the infiltrating immune cells. We found that Fas was markedly induced on cardiac myocytes with acute myocarditis. The induction of Fas expression on cardiac myocytes was confirmed *in vitro* by treatment with IFN -γ. *In vivo* administration of an anti-FasL mAb decreased myocardial inflammation as well as virus genomes in the heart. Myocardial inflammation was also decreased in Fas-deficient lpr/lpr and FasL-deficient gld/gld mice infected by CVB3 as compared with wild type [42]. This strongly suggested that Fas/FasL pathway played a critical role in the development of myocardial necrosis through activation of the infiltrating immune cells, rather than inducing apoptosis of cardiac myocytes.

CD40/CD40 ligand (CD40L): Another pathway of co-stimulatory molecules CD40, CD40L, which belong to the TNF receptor/ligand superfamily, is known to induce expression of B7 antigens and cytokine production by APCs, and to initiate T-cell-dependent antibody responses [43-45]. We found that CD40 was clearly induced on cardiac myocytes with acute myocarditis, and that the expression of CD40 on cardiac myocytes was induced by treatment with IFN-γ *in vitro*. We also found that the production of interleukin-6 by cultured cardiac myocytes was markedly enhanced by treatment with an anti-CD40 mAb *in vitro*. *In vivo* administration of an anti-CD40L mAb significantly decreased myocardial inflammation, indicating a critical role of CD40/CD40L pathway in the development of acute murine myocarditis [46].

CD30/CD30L, CD27/CD27L, OX40/OX40L, 4-1BB/4-1BBL: Other co-stimulatory molecules belonging to the TNF receptor/ligand superfamily include CD30/CD30L, CD27/CD27L, OX40/OX40L, and 4-1BB/4-1BBL [47, 48]. We again investigated the roles of these co-stimulatory molecules in the development of acute murine myocarditis [49]. Acute myocarditis caused by CVB3 clearly induced the expression of 4-1BBL and CD30L on cardiac myocytes *in vivo*, whereas CD27L and OX40L were constitutively expressed on cardiac myocytes. Induction of 4-1BBL and CD30L on cardiac myocytes was confirmed by treatment with IFN-γ *in vitro*. Anti-4-1BBL or -CD30L mAb along with IFN-γ significantly stimulated the production of interleukin-6 by cultured cardiac myocytes *in vitro*. Furthermore, *in vivo* administration of anti-4-1BBL mAb (but not other mAbs) significantly decreased myocardial inflammation, indicating the critical role of 4-1BB/4-1BBL pathway in the development of acute viral myocarditis. We found a persistent expression of CD40 and CD30L on cardiac myocytes in a murine model of chronic ongoing myocarditis as well [50].

4. Therapeutic interventions

1. *In vivo* antibody therapy

It is known that immunosuppressant therapy with corticosteroids or cyclosporin [51] may exacerbate acute viral myocarditis by enhancing virus titers. Godeny and Gauntt [3, 4] reported that depleting NK cells by injection of anti-asialo GM1 antiserum exacerbated murine viral myocarditis with increase in virus titers in the heart, indicating the protective role of NK cells against viral myocarditis by limiting virus replication. Therefore, nonspecific immunotherapies inhibiting virus-clearance seem to worsen the course of viral myocarditis, at least in the acute phase when virus genomes have not disappeared yet. We showed that immunomodulation therapy specifically targeting co-stimulatory molecules, such as ICAM-1 and FasL by *in vivo* administration of blocking mAbs, can decrease myocardial damage without inhibiting (or even enhancing) virus-clearance [20, 42]. We also showed that immunomodulation therapy targeting co-stimulatory molecules B7-1, CD40L, 4-1BBL, and PD-1 (with stimulating mAb) can significantly attenuate myocardial inflammation [25, 46, 49, 34]. Although we did not analyze the effects of these therapies on the virus-clearance in the heart, the protective effects against myocardial injury strongly suggested that immunomodulation therapies targeting these co-stimulatory molecules improve the course of myocarditis without inhibiting virus-clearance. The relative effects of immunomodulation therapies targeting co-stimulatory molecules is summarized in Figure 2. Recently, Fousteri et al. reported that *in vivo* administration of anti-OX40L mAb strongly reduced the inflammation of chronic phase of CVB3-induced murine myocarditis, supporting the role of these co-stimulatory molecules in progression to autoimmune phase [52].

2. IFNs

IFNs are among the most important antiviral agents, and are clinically used in hematological malignancy, autoimmune disorder, and viral infection such as hepatitis B and C. For viral myocarditis, the effectiveness of IFN-α A/D in a murine model of viral myocarditis was reported [53, 54]. Yamamoto et al. [55] analyzed the effects of IFN-γ and IFN-α/β by intranasal and intramuscular routes on murine viral myocarditis. The authors found that both IFN-γ and IFN-α/β by either route significantly increased the survival rate and that the effect of IFN-γ was significantly greater than that of IFN-α/β. The survival–prolonging effect of IFN-γ was confirmed even when started after virus inoculation. Furthermore, intranasal administration of IFN-γ significantly suppressed the virus replication and inflammation in the heart, which in turn dramatically improved the prognosis of acute murine viral myocarditis. The intranasal administration of IFN-γ offers a very useful antiviral therapy for acute myocarditis in clinical use.

3. TNF-α

TNF- α is another major cytokine known to be involved in viral myocarditis. Wada et al. [56] reported that survival rate of TNF- α-deficient mice with acute viral myocarditis was significantly lower than that of wild-type control mice, and *in vivo* administration of recombinant TNF- α improved the survival of TNF- α-deficient mice in a dose dependent manner. Although the authors speculated that TNF-α plays a protective role in acute viral myocarditis through leukocyte recruitment, it is unclear whether administration of TNF- α improves the survival of wild-type mice with acute viral myocarditis.

4. Angiotensin II receptor blockers (ARBs)

Angiotensin II has been shown to play an important role in the pathophysiology of various organs, especially the cardiovascular system. The effects of ARB on hypertension, congestive heart failure, and myocardial fibrosis have been well analyzed in human trials as well as animal models. The focus of interest is now directed to its pleiotropic effects especially on the inflammatory disorders. To investigate the effects of the ARB olmesartan on the cell-mediated myocardial injury involved in acute myocarditis, we analyzed the effects of olmesartan on the development of murine acute myocarditis caused by CVB3 [57]. We found that olmesartan

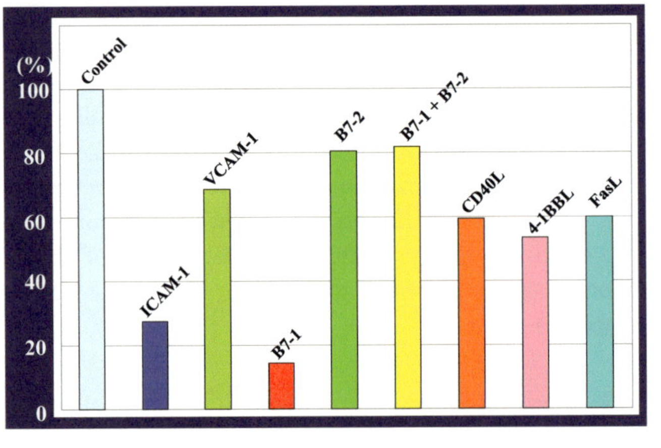

Figure 2. Summary of relative effects of immunomodulation therapies targeting co-stimulatory molecules in murine acute myocarditis.

http://dx.doi.org/10.5772/55165

significantly decreased myocardial inflammation as compared with control. Olmesartan also significantly decreased the expression of IFN-γ, FasL, inducible nitric oxide synthase (iNOS), perforin as well as CVB3 genomes in myocardial tissue, indicating that olmesartan suppressed activation of the infiltrating killer lymphocytes without inhibiting virus-clearance. This raises a possibility that olmesartan will reduce myocardial injury and improve prognosis of patients with acute myocarditis. Although we did not examine whether other ARBs have also protective effects against myocardial inflammation, there is a possibility that the prognosis of acute myocarditis patients receiving ARBs may be better than those not treated with ARBs.

5. Beta-adrenergic receptor blockers (β-blockers)

β-blockers, as well as angiotensin-converting enzyme inhibitors (ACEIs) and ARBs, have now been established as the therapy of heart failure. Especially, carvedilol, a non-selective β1, β2 (and less potent α1)-blocker, is known for its anti-oxidant properties [58]. In murine model of viral myocarditis, carvedilol was shown to attenuate the inflammation and improve left ventricular function through modulating the production of inflammatory cytokines and matrix metalloproteinases [59-61]. Because selective β1-blocker, metoprolol was much less effective, the cardioprotective effects of carvedilol may be due to pleiotropic effects as well as β-blocking effects, would be potentially useful in the treatment of patients with acute myocarditis.

6. Anti-virus therapy

Werk et al. [62] reported the effects of two anti-viral strategies, siRNA to degrade cytoplasmic CVB3 RNA, and a soluble variant of the coxsackievirus-adenovirus receptor fused to a human immunoglobulin (sCAR-Fc) to inhibit cellular uptake of CVB3. The authors demonstrated that combination therapy resulted in a strong synergistic inhibition of an ongoing virus infection. Because the study was done using a cell culture system, further study using an *in vivo* infection model is needed. Moreover, it is unknown whether the combination therapy is effective on patients with acute myocarditis who come to the hospital well after virus infection occurs.

Until now, not a few antiviral compounds have been developed and evaluated in clinical studies. WIN 63843 (pleconaril) is an orally bioavailable antiviral compound, which inhibits the binding of picornaviruses to the cell surface receptors and internalization of the viruses into the cell. In murine viral myocarditis caused by CVB3, pleconaril dramatically reduced the virus titer in the heart and increased the survival rate [63]. For other mechanism of antiviral activity, nitric oxide-releasing compounds such as glyceryl trinitrate (GTN) and isosorbide dinitrate (ISDN) were shown to inhibit proteinases 2A and 3C of CVB3, resulting in inhibition of viral replication and protecting the host cells from the cytopathic effects. Furthermore, GTN and ISDN significantly reduced the myocardial inflammation in murine model of viral myocarditis caused by CVB3 [64]. These antiviral therapeutics seem to be effective in the very early phase of viral myocarditis when viral replication actively occurs. However, in general, patients with acute myocarditis go to hospital after signs of inflammation have appeared when immune response to the virus-infected cells but not cytopathic effects of viruses mainly mediate myocardial injury. Therefore, the effectiveness of these antiviral therapeutics should be evaluated in clinical studies. On the other hand, Fousteri et al. reported that nasal administration of cardiac myosin-derived oligopeptides (CM-peptides) significantly reduced myocardial inflammation and mortality by enhancing regulatory T cells and IL-10 production in murine myocarditis caused by CVB3 [52]. However, the authors started the administration of CM-peptides before CVB3-infection. Because it is impossible to start the treatment at such timing clinically, efficiency of the therapy should be evaluated when started after the onset of inflammation.

7. Cell therapy

Mesenchymal stem cells (MSCs) are known to have anti-apoptotic, anti-fibrotic, pro-angiogenic, as well as immunomodulatory features. Linthout et al. [65] demonstrated that MSCs reduced CVB3-infected cardiomyocytes apoptosis and viral production in a nitric oxide-dependent manner *in vitro*, and MSCs required priming via IFN-γ to exert their protective effects. Furthermore, *in vivo* administration of MSCs in mice with CVB3-induced myocarditis improved cardiac function through reduction in cardiac apoptosis and myocardial injury. The authors also isolated and identified novel cardiac-derived cells from human cardiac biopsy specimen, that is cardiac-derived adherent proliferating cells (CAPs). CAPs have anti-apoptotic and immunomodulatory features similar to MSCs. Like MSCs, *in vivo* administration of CAPs in mice with CVB3-induced myocarditis improved cardiac function through reduction in cardiac apoptosis and virus proliferation [66].

8. MicroRNA

MicroRNAs (miRNAs) are small non-coding RNA molecules endogenously held by many species. It is known that miRNAs repress the expression of mRNAs by binding to 3 ' untranslated region of their target mRNAs. Corsten et al. [67] analyzed the profiles of miRNA expression in myocardial biopsy specimen from patients with acute myocarditis, and in myocardial tissue from myocarditis-susceptible and non-susceptible strain of mice with CVB3-induced acute myocarditis. They found that expression of microRNA-155, primarily localized in infiltrating cells, was consistently and strongly upregulated during acute myocarditis in both humans and susceptible mice. Inhibition of microRNA-155 by a systemically delivered locked nucleic acid (LNA)-anti-miRNA, a class of miRNA inhibitors, attenuated cardiac cell infiltration and myocardial damage in acute phase of murine myocarditis. MicroRNA-155 inhibition further improved cardiac function and reduced mortality of mice with viral myocarditis in later phase, offering a promising therapy against acute myocarditis. MicroRNA-122 is expressed in the liver, and is implicated as a key regulator of cholesterol and fatty-acid metabolism. Elmen et al. [68] first demonstrated using African green monkeys that *in vivo* administration of LNA-anti-microRNA-122 resulted in long-lasting decrease in plasma cholesterol levels without any toxicities. For anti-microRNA therapy against viral infection in primates, Lanford et al. [69] reported that treatment of chimpanzees chronically infected with hepatitis C virus with LNA-anti-microRNA-122 resulted in long-lasting suppression of viremia and improvement of liver pathology with safety profile. Successful study in primates against virus infection common to a human disease may strongly support clinical trials in patients with hepatitis C virus infection as well as acute myocarditis.

http://dx.doi.org/10.5772/55165

Author details

Yoshinori Seko

Address all correspondence to: sekoyosh-tky@umin.ac.jp

Division of Cardiovascular Medicine, The Institute for Adult Diseases, Asahi Life Foundation, 2-2-6 Nihonbashibakurocho, Chuo-ku, Tokyo, Japan

References

[1] Woodruff JF: Viral myocarditis: A review. *Am J Pathol* 1980;101:427-484.

[2] Guthrie M, Lodge PAA, Huber SA: Cardiac injury in myocarditis induced by coxsackievirus group B type 3 in BALB/c mice is mediated by Lyt 2+ cytolytic lymphocytes. *Cell Immunol* 1984;88:558-567.

[3] Godeny EK, Gauntt CJ: Involvement of natural killer cells in coxsackievirus B3-induced murine myocarditis. *J Immunol* 1986;137:1695-1702.

[4] Godeny EK, Gauntt CJ: Murine natural killer cells limit coxsackievirus B3 replication. *J Immunol* 1987;139:913-918.

[5] Seko Y, Shinkai Y, Kawasaki A, Yagita H, Okumura K, Takaku F, Yazaki Y: Expression of perforin in infiltrating cells in murine hearts with acute myocarditis caused by Coxsackievirus B3. *Circulation* 1991;84:788-795.

[6] Shinkai Y, Takio K, Okumura K: Homology of perforin to the ninth component of complement (C9). *Nature* 1988;334:525-527.

[7] Young JDE: Killing of target cells by lymphocytes: A mechanistic view. *Physiol Rev* 1989;69:250-314.

[8] Young LHY, Klavinskis LS, Oldstone MBA, Young JDE: *In vivo* expression of perforin by CD8+ lymphocytes during acute viral infection. *J Exp Med* 1989;169:2159-2171.

[9] Seko Y, Shinkai Y, Kawasaki A, Yagita H, Okumura K, Yazaki Y: Evidence of perforin-mediated cardiac myocyte injury in acute murine myocarditis caused by Coxsackievirus B3. *J Pathol* 1993;170:53-58.

[10] Seko Y, Ishiyama S, Nishikawa T, Kasajima T, Hiroe M, Kagawa N, Osada K, Suzuki S, Yagita H, Okumura K, Yazaki Y: Restricted usage of T cell receptor Vα-Vβ genes in infiltrating cells in the hearts of patients with acute myocarditis and dilated cardiomyopathy.*J Clin Invest* 1995;96:1035-1041.

[11] Gebhard JR, Perry CM, Harkins S, Lane T, Mena I, Asensio V rie C, Campbell IL, Whitton JL: Coxsackievirus B3-induced myocarditis. Perforin exacerbates disease, but plays no detectable role in virus clearance. *Am J Pathol* 1998;153:417-428.

[12] Seko Y, Yagita H, Okumura K, Yazaki Y: T-cell receptor Vβ gene expression in infiltrating cells in murine hearts with acute myocarditis caused by Coxsackievirus B3. *Circulation* 1994;89:2170-2175.

[13] Ploegh HL, Orr HT, Strominger JL: Major histocompatibility antigens : The human (HLA-A, -B, -C) and murine (H-2K, H-2D) class I molecules. *Cell* 1981;24:287-299.

[14] Kaufman JF, Auffray C, Korman AJ, Shackelford, DA, Strominger JL: The class II molecules of the human and murine major histocompatibility complex. *Cell* 1984;36:1-13.

[15] Daar AS, Fuggle SV, Fabre JW, Ting A, Morris PJ: The detailed distribution of HLA-A, B, C antigens in normal human organs. *Transplantation* 1984;38:287-292.

[16] Daar AS, Fuggle SV, Fabre JW, Ting A, Morris PJ: The detailed distribution of MHC class II antigens in normal human organs. *Transplantation* 1984;38:293-298.

[17] Seko Y, Tsuchimochi H, Nakamura T, Okumura K, Naito S, Imataka K, Fujii J, Takaku F, Yazaki Y: Expression of major histocompatibility complex class I antigen in murine ventricular myocytes infected with coxsackievirus B3. *Circ Res* 1990;67:360-367.

[18] Mueller DL, Jenkins MK, Schwartz RH: Clonal expansion versus functional clonal inactivation: a co-stimulatory signaling pathway determines the outcome of T cell antigen receptor occupancy. *Annu Rev Immunol* 1989;7:445-480.

[19] Wawryk SO, Novotny JR, Wicks IP, Wilkinson D, Maher D, Salvaris E, Welch K, Fecondo J, Boyd AW: The role of LFA-1/ICAM-1 interaction in human leukocyte homing and adhesion. *Immunol Rev* 1989;108:135-161.

[20] Seko Y, Matsuda H, Kato K, Hashimoto Y, Yagita H, Okumura K, Yazaki Y: Expression of intercellular adhesion molecule-1 in murine hearts with acute myocarditis caused by Coxsackievirus B3. *J Clin Invest* 1993;91:1327-1336.

[21] Seko Y, Yagita H, Okumura K, Yazaki Y: Expression of vascular cell adhesion molecule-1 in murine hearts with acute myocarditis caused by Coxsackievirus B3. *J Pathol* 1996;180:450-454.

[22] Azuma M, Ito D, Yagita H, Okumura K, Phillips JH, Lanier LL, Somoza C: B70 antigens is a second ligand for CTLA-4 and CD28. *Nature* 1993;366:76-79.

[23] Hathcock KS, Laszlo G, Dickler HB, Bradshaw J, Linsley P, Hodes RJ: Identification of an alternative CTLA-4ligand co-stimulatory for T cell activation. *Science* 1993;262:905-907.

[24] Freeman GJ, Gribben JG, Boussiotis VA, Ng JW, Restivo VA Jr, Lombard LA, Gray GS, Nadler LM: Cloning of B7-2: a CTLA-4 counter-receptor that costimulates human T cell proliferation. *Science* 1993;262:909-911.

[25] Seko Y, Takahashi N, Azuma M, Yagita H, Okumura K, Yazaki Y: Effects of *In vivo* administration of anti-7-1/B7-2 monoclonal antibodies on murine acute myocarditis caused by coxsackievirus B3. *Circ Res* 1998;82:613-618.

[26] Seko Y, Takahashi N, Yagita H, Okumura K, Azuma M, Yazaki Y: Effects of *In vivo* administration of anti-7-1/B7-2 monoclonal antibodies on the survival of mice with chronic ongoing myocarditis caused by coxsackievirus B3. *J Pathol* 1999;188:107-112.

[27] Seko Y, Takahashi N, Ishiyama S, Nishikawa T, Kasajima T, Hiroe M, et al.: Expression of co-stimulatory molecules B7-1, B7-2, and CD40 in the heart of patients with acute myocarditis and dilated cardiomyopathy. *Circulation* 1998;97:637-639.

[28] Frisancho-Kiss S, Nyland JF, Davis SE, Barrett MA, Gatewood SJ, Njoku DB, Cihakova D, Silbergeld EK, Rose NR, Fairweather D: Cutting edge: T cell Ig mucin-3 reduces inflammatory heart disease by increasing CTLA-4 during innate immunity. J Immunol 2006;176:6411-6415.

[29] Love VA, Grabie N, Duramad P, Stavrakis G, Sharpe A, Lichtman A: CTLA-4 ablation and interleukin-12–driven differentiation synergistically augment cardiac pathogenicity of cytotoxic T lymphocytes. *Circ Res* 2007;101:248-257.

[30] Ishida Y, Agata Y, Shibahara K, Honjo T: Induced expression of PD-1, a novel member of the immunoglobulin gene superfamily, upon programmed cell death. *EMBO J* 1992;11:3887-3895.

[31] Nishimura H, Honjo T: PD-1: an inhibitory immunoreceptor involved in peripheral tolerance. *Trends Immunol* 2001;22:265-268.

[32] Freeman GJ, Long AJ, Iwai Y, Bourque K, Chernova T, Nishimura H, et al.: Engagement of the PD-1 immunoinhibitory receptor by a novel B7 family member leads to negative regulation for lymphocyte activation. *J Exp Med* 200;192:1027-1034.

[33] Latchman Y, Wood CR, Chernova T, Chaudhary D, Borde M, Chernova I, et al.: PD-L2 is a second ligand for PD-1 and inhibits T cell activation. *Nat Immunol* 2001;2:261-268.

[34] Seko Y, Yagita H, Okumura K, Azuma M, Nagai R: Roles of programmed death-1 (PD-1)/PD-1 ligands pathway in the development of murine acute myocarditis caused by coxsackievirus B3. *Cardiovasc Res* 2007;75:158-167.

[35] Yonehara S, Ishii A,Yonehara M: A cell-killing monoclonal antibody (anti-Fas) to a cell surface antigen co-downregulated with the receptor of tumor necrosis factor. *J Exp Med*1989;169:1747-1756.

[36] Trauth BC, Klas C, Peters AM, Matzku S, Möller P, Falk W, et al.: Monoclonal antibody-mediated tumor regression by induction of apoptosis. *Science*1989;245:301-305.

[37] Itoh N, Yonehara S, Ishii A, Yonehara M, Mizushima S, Sameshima M, et al.: The polypeptide encoded by the cDNA for human cell surface antigen Fas can mediate apoptosis. *Cell*1991;66:233-243.

[38] Suda T, Takahashi T, Golstein P, Nagata S: Molecular cloning and expression of the Fas ligand: a novel member of the tumor necrosis factor family. *Cell* 1993;75:1169-1178.

[39] Rouvier E, Luciani M-F, Goldstein P: Fas involvement in Ca^{2+}-independent T cell-mediated cytotoxicity. *J Exp Med*1993;177:195-200.

[40] Hanabuchi S, Koyanagi M, Kawasaki A, Shinohara N, Matsuzawa A, Nishimura Y, et al.: Fas and its ligand in a general mechanism of T cell-mediated cytotoxicity. *Proc Natl Acad Sci USA* 1994;91:4930-4934.

[41] Arase H, Arase N, Saito T: Fas-mediated cytotoxicity by freshly isolated natural killer cells. *J Exp Med* 1995;181:1235-1238.

[42] Seko Y, Kayagaki N, Seino K, Yagita H, Okumura K, Nagai R: Role of Fas/FasL pathway in the activation of infiltrating cells in murine acute myocarditis caused by coxsackievirus B3. *J Am Coll Cardiol* 2002;39:1399-1403.

[43] Caux C, Massacrier C, Vanbervliet B, Dubois B, Van-Kooten C, Durand I, Banchereau J: Activation of human dendritic cells through CD40 cross-linking. *J Exp Med* 1994;180:1263-1272.

[44] Ranheim EA, Kipps TJ: Activated T cells induce expression of B7/BB1 on normal or leukemic B cells through a CD40-dependent signal. *J Exp Med* 1993;177:925-935.

[45] Kelsall BL, Stuber E, Neurath M, Strober W: Interleukin-12 production by dendritic cells: the role of CD40-CD40L interactions in Th1 T-cell responses. *Ann NY Acad Sci* 1996;795:116-126.

[46] Seko Y, Takahashi N, Azuma M, Yagita H, Okumura K, Yazaki Y: Expression of co-stimulatory molecule CD40 in murine heart with acute myocarditis and reduction inflammation by treatment with anti-CD40L/B7-1 monoclonal antibodies. *Circ Res* 1998;83:463-469.

[47] Smith CA, Farrah T, Goodwin RG: The TNF receptor superfamily of cellular and viral proteins: activation, costimulation, and death. *Cell* 1994;76:959-962.

[48] Gruss HJ, Dower SK: Tumor necrosis factor ligand superfamily: involvement in the pathology of malignant lymphomas. *Blood* 1995;85:3378-3404.

[49] Seko Y, Takahashi N, Oshima H, Shimozato O, Akiba H, Takeda K, et al.: Expression of tumor necrosis factor (TNF) ligand superfamily co-stimulatory molecules CD30L,

CD27L, OX40L, and 4-1BBL in murine hearts with acute myocarditis caused by coxsackievirus B3. *J Pathol* 2001;195:593-603.

[50] Seko Y, Takahashi N, Oshima H, Shimozato O, Akiba H, Kobata T, et al.: Expression of tumor necrosis factor (TNF) receptor/ligand superfamily co-stimulatory molecules CD40, CD30L, CD27L, and OX40 in murine hearts with chronic ongoing myocarditis caused by coxsackievirus B3. *J Pathol* 1999;188:423-430.

[51] O'Connell JB, Reap EA, Robinson JA: The effects of cyclosporine on acute murine Coxsackie B3 myocarditis. *Circulation*1986;73:353-359.

[52] Fousteri G, Dave A, Morin B, Omid S, Croft M, von Herrath MG: Nasal cardiac myosin peptide treatment and OX40 blockade protect mice from acute and chronic virally-induced myocarditis. *J Autoimmun* 2011;36:210-220.

[53] Weck PK, Rinderknecht E, Estell DA, Stebbing N: Antiviral activity of bacteria-derived human alpha interferons against encephalomyocarditis virus infection of mice. *Infect Immun* 1982;35:660-665.

[54] Matsumori A, Crumpacker CS, Abelmann WH: Prevention of viral myocarditis with recombinant human leukocyte interferon α A/D in murine model. *J Am Coll Cardiol* 1987;9:1320-1325.

[55] Yamamoto N, Shibamori M, Ogura M, Seko Y, Kikuchi M: Effects of intranasal administration of recombinant murine interferon-γ on murine acute myocarditis caused by encephalomyocarditis virus. *Circulation* 1998;97:1017-1023.

[56] Wada H, Saito K, Kanda K, Kobayashi I, Fujii H, Fujigaki S, Maekawa N, Takatsu H, Fujiwara H, Sekikawa K, Seishima M: Tumor necrosis factor-α (TNF-α) plays a protective role in acute viral myocarditis in mice : a study using mice lacking TNF- α. *Circulation* 2001;103:743-749.

[57] Seko Y: Effect of the angiotensin II receptor blocker olmesartan on the development of murine acute myocarditis caused by coxsackievirus B3. *Clin Sci* 2006;110:379-386.

[58] Book WM: Carvedilol: a nonselective beta blocking agent with antioxidant properties. *Congest Heart Fail* 2002;8:173-177.

[59] Nishio R, Shioi T, Sasayama S, Matsumori A: Carvedilol increases the production of interleukin-12 and interferon-gamma and improves the survival of mice infected with the encephalomyocarditis virus. *J Am Coll Cardiol* 2003; 41:340-345.

[60] Tschöpe C, Westermann D, Steendijk P, Noutsias M, Rutschow S, Weitz A, Schwimmbeck PL, Schultheiss HP, Pauschinger M: Hemodynamic characterization of left ventricular function in experimental coxsackieviral myocarditis: effects of carvedilol and metoprolol. *Eur J Pharmacol* 2004;491:173-179.

[61] Pauschinger M, Rutschow S, Chandrasekharan K, Westermann D, Weitz A, Peter Schwimmbeck L, Zeichhardt H, Poller W, Noutsias M, Li J, Schultheiss HP, Tschope C: Carvedilol improves left ventricular function in murine coxsackievirus-induced

acute myocarditis association with reduced myocardial interleukin-1beta and MMP-8 expression and a modulated immune response. *Eur J Heart Fail* 2005;7:444-452.

[62] Werk D, Pinkert S, Heim A, Zeichhardt H, Grunert HP, Poller W, Erdmann VA, Fechner H, Kurreck J: Combination of soluble coxsackievirus-adenovirus receptor and anti-coxsackievirus siRNAs exerts synergistic antiviral activity against coxsackievirus B3. Antiviral Res 2009; 83:298-306.

[63] Pevear DC, Tull TM, Seipel ME, Groarke JM: Activity of pleconaril against enteroviruses. *Antimicrob Agents Chemother* 1999;43: 2109-2115.

[64] Zell R, Markgraf R, Schmidtke M, Gorlach M, Stelzner A, Henke A, Sigusch HH, Gluck, B: Nitric oxide donors inhibit the coxsackievirus B3 proteinases 2A and 3C *in vitro*, virus production in cells, and signs of myocarditis in virus-infected mice. *Med Microbiol Immunol* 2004;193:91-100.

[65] van Linthout S, Savvatis K, Miteva K, Peng J, Ringe J, Warstat K,C. Schmidt-Lucke C, Sittinger M, Schultheiss HP, Tschope C: Mesenchymal stem cells improve murine acute coxsackievirus B3-induced myocarditis. *Eur Heart J* 2011;32:2168–2178.

[66] Miteva K, Haag M, Peng J, Savvatis K, Becher PM, Seifert M, Warstat K, Westermann D, Ringe J, Sittinger M, Schultheiss HP, Tschöpe C, van Linthout S: Human cardiac-derived adherent proliferating cells reduce murine acute Coxsackievirus B3-induced myocarditis. PLoS One 2011;6:e28513.

[67] Corsten MF, Papageorgiou A, Verhesen W, Carai P, Lindow M, Obad S, Summer G, Coort SL, Hazebroek M, van Leeuwen R, Gijbels MJ, Wijnands E, Biessen EA, De Winther MP, Stassen FR, Carmeliet P, Kauppinen S, Schroen B, Heymans S: MicroRNA profiling identifies microRNA-155 as an adverse mediator of cardiac injury and dysfunction during acute viral myocarditis. *Circ Res* 2012;111:415-425.

[68] Elmen J, Lindow M, Schutz S, Lawrence M, Petri A, Obad S, Lindholm M, Hedtjarn M, Hansen HF, Berger U, Gullans S, Kearney P, Sarnow P, Straarup EM, Kauppinen S: LNA-mediated microRNA silencing in non-human primates. *Nature* 2008;452:896–899.

[69] Lanford RE, Hildebrandt-Eriksen ES, Petri A, Persson R, Lindow M, Munk ME, Kauppinen S, Ørum H: Therapeutic silencing of microRNA-122 in primates with chronic hepatitis C virus infection. *Science* 2010; 327: 198-201.

Section 3

Diagnosis

Chapter 4

Endomyocardial Biopsy: A Clinical Research Tool and a Useful Diagnostic Method

Julián González, Francisco Salgado,
Francisco Azzato, Giuseppe Ambrosio and
Jose Milei

Additional information is available at the end of the chapter

http://dx.doi.org/10.5772/54399

1. Introduction

The routine indication of endomyocardial biopsy (EMB) in myocarditis has long been a matter of debate [1]. Although always claimed as the ultimate diagnostic tool for myocarditis, its low sensitivity, low availability, high cost, and the inherent risks of an invasive procedure have led many physicians to avoid performing it. Yet, at present EMB continues to be the "gold standard" for the diagnosis of myocarditis [2].

Since its introduction in the early 1960s by Sakakibara and Konno many improvements have been made in the technique and some progress has been made in the analysis of the samples. The introduction of the Dallas Criteria [3] in 1986 was the first effort to make histological diagnosis more consistent, but still they have a very low sensitivity and lack prognostic value in many clinical studies [4-7].

After the Dallas criteria, the use of immunohistochemistry to better identify mononuclear cells infiltrating myocardial tissue added significant sensitivity to histological diagnosis [8, 9]. Also, introduction of polymerase chain reaction (PCR) applied to isolation of viral genomes from EMB samples became a promising tool. Both proved to carry prognostic value in some studies, but results have been not consistent in all publications.

Moreover, development of noninvasive methods to assess myocardial injury in myocarditis, particularly magnetic resonance image (MRI), provides a very interesting alternative to EMB, although some authors suggest that they may be complementary [10].

In this chapter we will review the most relevant evidence of the clinical usefulness of EMB and all these developing techniques.

2. Technical issues on endomyocardial biopsies

The first approach to obtain tissue samples from the heart was proposed in the 1950s by Vim and Silverman by using a needle introduced through a limited thoracotomy. The high incidence of pneumothorax and cardiac tamponade made this technique not accepted [11]. It was in 1962 that for the first time Sakakibara and Konno reported their technique of EMB introducing the bioptome in order to sample the endocardium [12]. After developmentof the bioptome, many improvements have been made in terms of flexibility and maneuverability, making the procedure safer and easier.

The possibility of peripheral vein access made the right ventricle the most attractive site for sampling, especially the interventricular septum because it is thicker than the right ventricular free wall and it is located in the natural path of blood flow [11]. Anyway, if needed, the left ventricle may be reached through the femoral artery and across the aortic valve [13].

According to current recommendations of the International Society of Heart and Lung Transplantation [14] and the American Heart Association, American College of Cardiology and European Society of Cardiology [2] a minimum of 4 -5 samples of 1 – 2 mm^3 in size should be collected at room temperature to prevent contraction band artifacts. Additional samples may be taken if special procedures are required as immunohistochemistry (IHC), transmission electron microscopy, and/or polymerase chain reaction.

Complications of EMB have been prospectively studied by Decker et al. [15] in 546 consecutive procedures. The overall complications rate was 6%, 2.7% related to sheath insertion and 3.3% related to the biopsy procedure itself. Perforation was observed in only 3 patients (0.5%) with 2 deaths attributable to perforations (0.3%). The detailed report is summarized in table 1.

Related to Sheath Insertion = 15 (2.7%)
Arterial puncture during local anesthesia = 12 (2%)
Vasovagal reaction = 2 (0.4%)
Prolonged venous oozing after sheath removal = 1 (0.2%)
Biopsy Procedure = 18 (3.3%)
Arrhythmias = 6 (1.1%)
Conduction abnormalities = 5 (1%)
Pain without perforation = 4 (0.7%)
Perforation = 3(0.5%), 2 patients died (0.3%)

Table 1. Complications of EMB (Deckers et al. [15])

http://dx.doi.org/10.5772/54399

3. Current recommendations for the use of endomyocardial biopsies

In an attempt to better determine the clinical use of EMB, a committee of experts from the American Heart Association, the American College of Cardiologists and the European Society of Cardiology developed a consensus statement about when EMB was to be used in 14 clinical scenarios [2]. It is remarkable that in only 2 of those scenarios the recommendation reaches recommendation level I. Table 2 summarizes the 14 clinical situations, the level of recommendation, and evidence for the use and clinical value of EBM.

Nº	Clinical Scenario	EMB usefulness	Level of recom.	Level of evid.
1	New-onset heart failure of <2 weeks' duration associated with a normal-size or dilated left ventricle and hemodynamic compromise	Distinguish between lymphocytic myocarditis (good prognosis) and GCM or NEM that require immunosupressant treatment.	I	B
2	New-onset heart failure of 2 weeks' to 3 months' duration associated with dilated left ventricle and new-onset ventricular arrhythmias, second- or third-degree heart block, or failure to respond to usual care within 1 to 2 weeks	Distinguish between lymphocytic myocarditis (good prognosis) and GCM that requires immunosupressant treatment.	I	B
3	Heart failure of >3 months' duration associated with dilated left ventricle and new-onset ventricular arrhythmias, second- or third-degree heart block, or failure to respond to usual care within 1 to 2 weeks	Cardiac sarcoidosis is a special differential diagnosis in this setting. Sarcoidosis responds very well to corticosteroid treatment. GCM is also a possibility in this scenario.	IIa	C
4	Heart failure associated with a DCM of any duration associated with suspected allergic reaction and/or eosinophilia	Detect HSM and stop offending medication and start high dose corticosteroids.	IIa	C
5	Heart failure associated with suspected anthracycline cardiomyopathy	Although anthracycline toxicity can be detected by means of noninvasive test, EMB has better sensitivity to detect earlier stages and stop offending drug earlier. Requires TEM.	IIa	C
6	Heart failure associated with unexplained restrictive cardiomyopathy	Although a great progress has been made in the use of noninvasive tests such as CMR in the assessment of restrictive	IIa	C

Nº	Clinical Scenario	EMB usefulness	Level of recom.	Level of evid.
		cardiomyopathy, EMB still remains the only diagnostic tool for many of them.		
7	Suspected cardiac tumors	When diagnosis is not possible through other methods. Not recommended in typical myxoma because of embolization risk.	IIa	C
8	Unexplained cardiomyopathy in children	Differential diagnosis	IIa	C
9	New-onset heart failure of 2 weeks' to 3 months' duration associated with a dilated left ventricle, without new-onset ventricular arrhythmias or second- or third-degree heart block, that responds to usual care within 1 to 2 weeks	Seldom GCM can be diagnosed in this setting. EMB should not be performed routinely.	IIb	B
10	Heart failure of >3 months' duration associated with a dilated left ventricle, without new ventricular arrhythmias or second- or third-degree heart block, that responds to usual care within 1 to 2 weeks	In recent trials patients showing enhanced expression of HLA molecules in EMB had some benefit from immunosuppressant therapy. Hemochromatosis may be a differential diagnosis in this setting.	IIb	C
11	Heart failure associated with unexplained HCM	Some entities, specially infiltrating diseases that can thicken heart walls, can be diagnosed with EMB (Pompe's and Fabry's diseases, amyloidosis).	IIb	C
12	Suspected ARVD/C	Rarely needed because CMR generally establishes the diagnosis.	IIb	C
13	Unexplained ventricular arrhythmias	Generally shows myocarditis or nonspecific findings.	IIb	C
14	Unexplained atrial fibrillation	Not recommended	III	C

CRM, Cardiac Magnetic Resonance; DCM, Dilated Cardiomyopathy; GCM, Giant Cell Myocarditis; HSM, Hypersensitivity Myocarditis; NEM, Necrotizing Eosinophilic Myocarditis; TEM, Transmission Electron Microscopy.

Table 2. Clinical Recommendations for the Use of EMB [2].

4. The anatomopathological picture of different types of myocarditis

We will briefly describe the pathological features of the main pathologies cited in this chapter that constitute the differential diagnosis of lymphocytic myocarditis:

http://dx.doi.org/10.5772/54399

- Lymphocytic myocarditis
- Giant cell myocarditis
- Sarcoidosis
- Hypersensitivity myocarditis
- Eosinophilic myocarditis

4.1. Lymphocytic myocarditis

The pathological picture of lymphocytic myocarditis is the infiltration of myocardium by activated T lymphocytes, with or without signs of myocyte injury, as illustrated by the EMB sample of a patient with cytomegalovirus (CMV) myocarditis shown in figures 1-3. Figure 3 also shows the characteristic nuclear inclusions of CMV infection. Histological findings are generally diffuse but may be focal in nature (figure 4) making multiple samples and immunohistochemistry necessary for greater diagnostic accuracy.

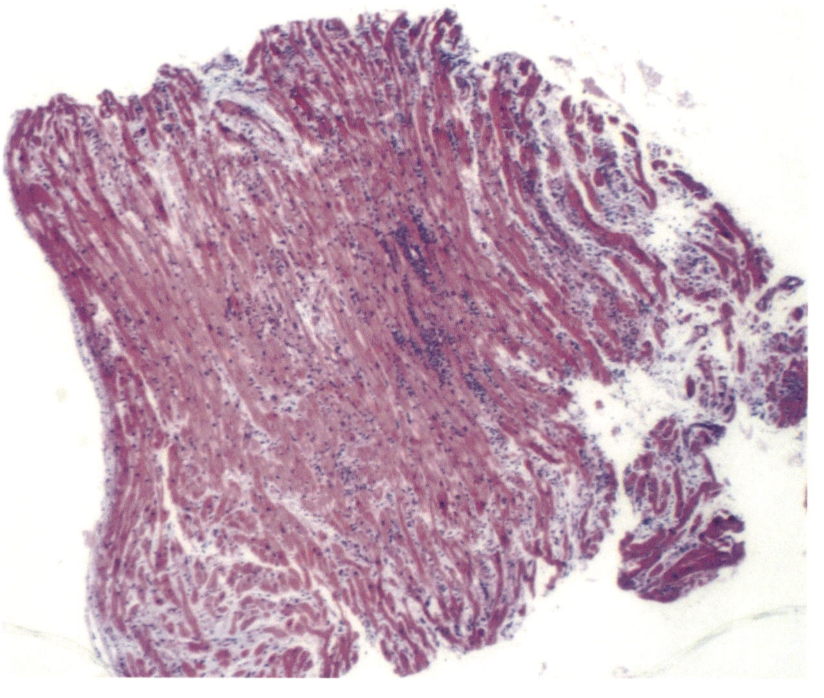

Figure 1. Myocarditis. Endomyocardial biopsy demonstrating a diffuse infiltration of lymphocytes. H-E. 40 X.

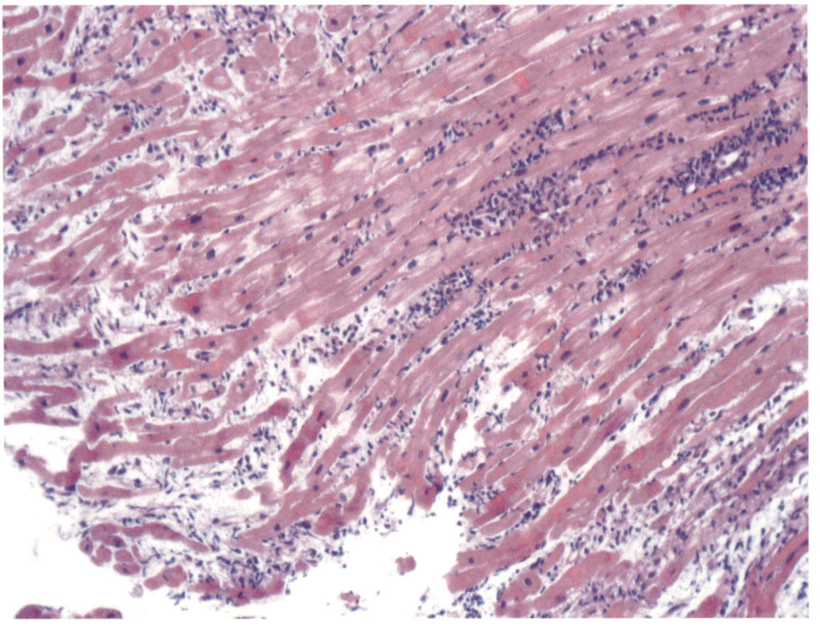

Figure 2. Myocarditis. Biopsy sample of the case illustrated in Figure 1. A dense infiltrate of lymphocytes and myocyte necrosis isevident. H-E- 100X.

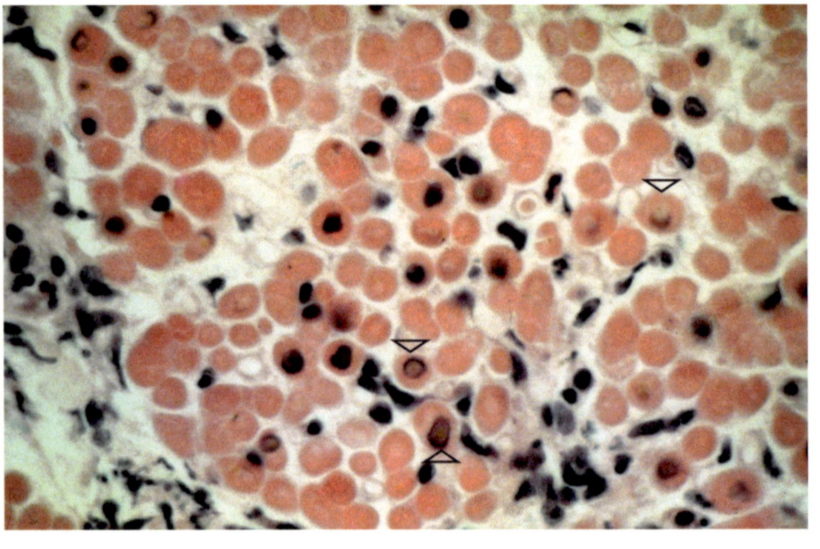

Figure 3. Myocarditis. Biopsy sample of the case illustrated in Figures 1 and 2. Lymphocytic myocarditis by cytomegalovirus infection. Note the characteristic "owl's eye" nuclear inclusions (arrows). H-E. 400X

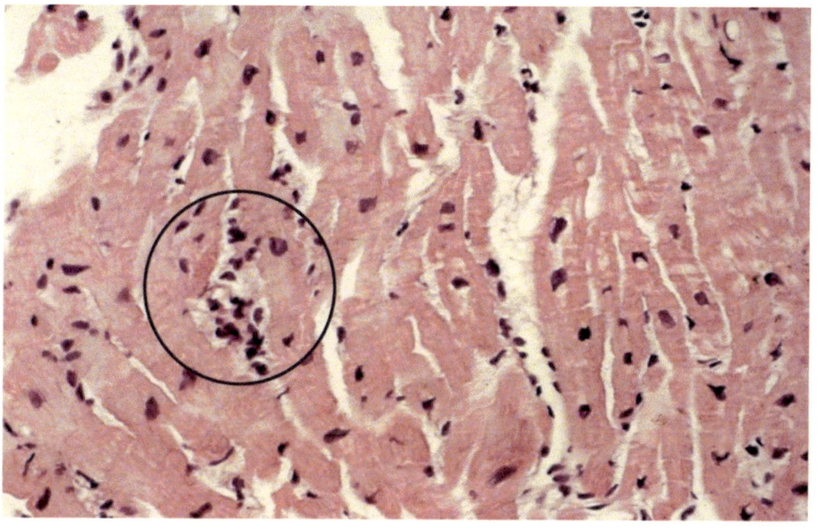

Figure 4. Focal myocarditis. Inflammation is quite focal. Note necrotic myocytes infiltrated by lymphocytes (circle) H-E 200X.

In order to better standardize histological diagnosis, Dallas criteria have been developed (table 3), for first and subsequent biopsies. **Active myocarditis** is defined as the presence of lymphocytes infiltrating myocardium plus evidence of myocyte injury (excluding contraction bands, a common artifact in EMB samples). **Borderline myocarditis** is defined as milder infiltrates without evidence of myocyte injury.

For subsequent biopsies, **ongoing** myocarditis, **resolving** (healing) **myocarditis** (figure 5) and **resolved** (healed) **myocarditis** categories have been created if infiltrates are the same as first biopsy, less than the first biopsy or have disappeared respectively.

First biopsy
Active myocarditis, with or without fibrosis
Borderline myocarditis
No myocarditis
Subsequent biopsy
Ongoing (persistent) myocarditis, with or without fibrosis
Healing (resolving) myocarditis, with or without fibrosis
Healed (resolved) myocarditis, with or without fibrosis

Table 3. Dallas criteria for the diagnosis of myocarditis

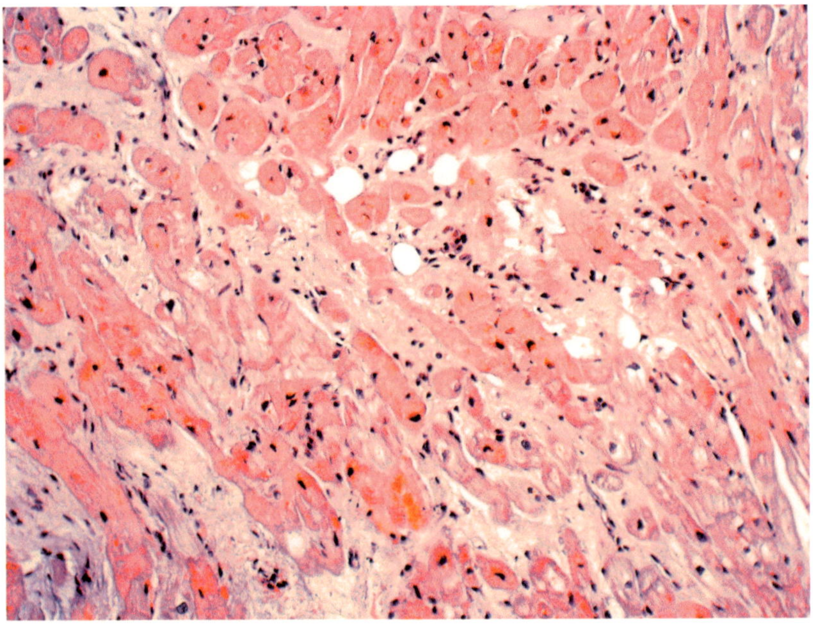

Figure 5. Healing myocarditis. Diffuse lymphocytic infiltrate is mingled with interstitial fibrosis. Note the scattered atrophic myocytes. H-E 200X.

4.2. Giant Cell Myocarditis (GCM)

This specific form of myocarditis of unknown cause is particularly aggressive with a high mortality. Extensive myocyte necrosis with an intensive infiltrate of lymphocytes, plasma cells and eosinophils are seen. The most striking characteristic, which names the disease, is the presence of giant multinucleated cells in the borders of necrotic areas (figure 6). Multinucleated cells are originated from macrophages. The most abundant cells in the remaining infiltrates are CD8+ T-lymphocytes. The main differential diagnosis of GCM is sarcoidosis, which is differentiated for:

- Eosinophils are abundant in GCM and absent in sarcoidosis
- Fibrotic scarring is more prominent in sarcoidosis
- No granulomas are seen un GCM
- Sarcoidosis may affectepicardium, never affected by GCM

http://dx.doi.org/10.5772/54399

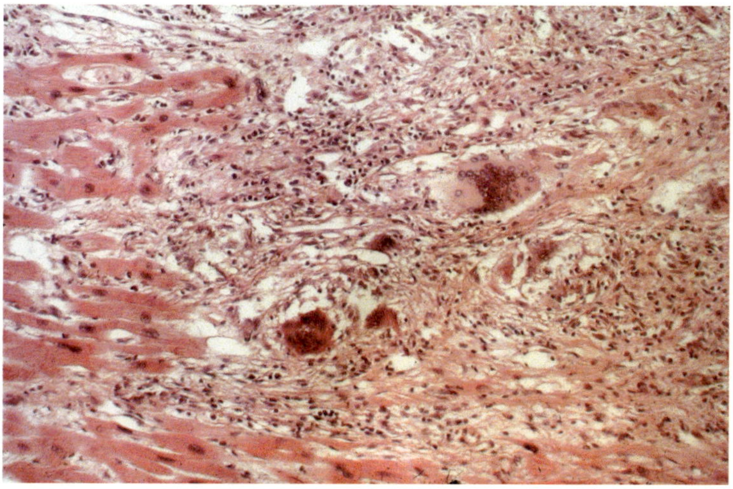

Figure 6. Giant cell myocarditis. A dense infiltrate of lymphocytes with prominent giant cells isobserved. Note the absence of well-established granulomas. H-E 200X.

4.3. Sarcoidosis

Sarcoidosis is a systemic disease that may affect the myocardium. The presence of granulomas on EMBs may reach 20% of cases. The compromise is patchy and EMBs may be negative. Non-caseificating granulomas consisting of histiocytes, giant cells, lymphocytes and plasma cells are the most prominent feature of the disease. Focal infiltrates of lymphocytes are seen, but they lack eosinophils seen in GCM. Patchy fibrosis is also a frequent finding (figure 7).

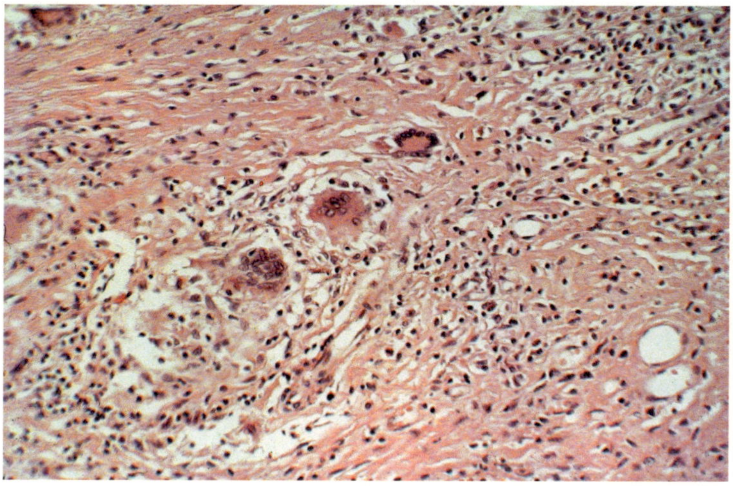

Figure 7. Sarcoidosis. Endomyocardial biopsy demonstrates a well-established, non-necrotizing granuloma. Giant cells are evident. H-E 200X.

4.4. Hypersensitivity myocarditis

Although not very common, hypersensitivity to drugs may involve the myocardium. The suspicion of this entity should arise when a patient presents with acute heart failure in the context of a hypersensitivity reaction to a drug. Tissue samples show a chronic perivascular infiltrates with lymphocytes, macrophages and plasma cells, with a prominence of eosinophils. Myocyte injury may be seen but is not a prominent feature. Fibrosis is absent.

4.5. Eosinophilic myocarditis

Myocarditis may be present up to in 25% of patients with hypereosinophilic syndrome. Extensive infiltration with eosinophils is present in this type of myocarditis (figure 8) but two distinctive features help distinguishing it from hypersensitivity myocarditis: the presence of myocyte necrosis and the presence of intracavitary thrombi containing eosinophils, which can also be seen in the lumen of intramyocardial coronary vessels.

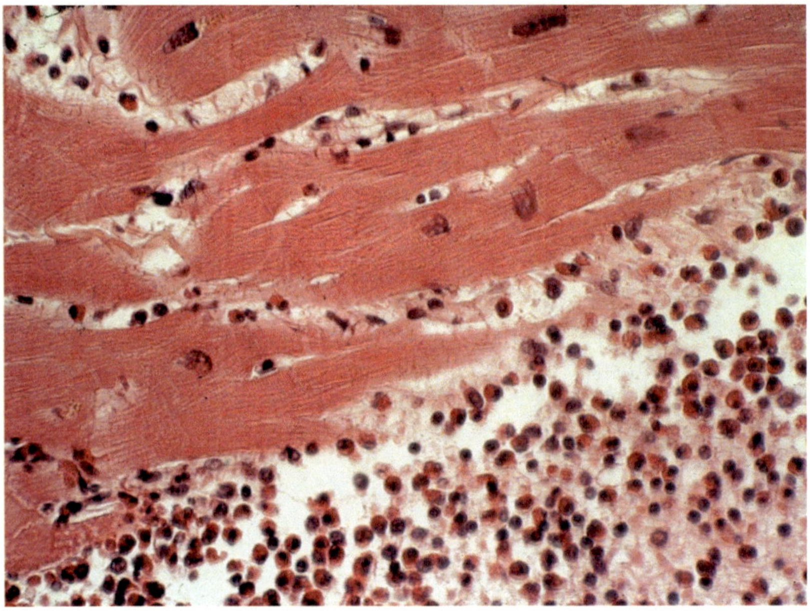

Figure 8. Hypereosinophilia. The interstitial infiltrate is suggestive of hypersensitivity myocarditis. H-E 200X

http://dx.doi.org/10.5772/54399

5. The role of endomyocardial biopsy in the management of myocarditis

Endomyocardial biopsy is still considered the "gold standard" for diagnosis of viral myocarditis. The use of Dallas criteria, although questioned, remains almost universal. The development of IHC and PCR for processing EMB samples widened its usefulness.

5.1. The rise, decline and validity of the Dallas criteria

The Dallas criteria for histopathological diagnosis of myocarditis were introduced in 1986 [3] in the intent of standardizing the way in which EMB would be analyzed and became, since then, a "gold standard" for the definitive diagnosis of myocarditis.

As previously stated, **active myocarditis** was defined as the presence of inflammatory infiltrates associated with myocardial injury not characteristic of ischemic heart disease, and **borderline myocarditis** was defined as a les intensive infiltrate without evidence of myocyte damage.

Furthermore, most clinical investigation on myocarditis have used the Dallas criteria as the main inclusion criteria [16]. The main weakness of Dallas criteria is low sensitivity (about 25%) to detect infiltrates in myocardial samples, mainly due to: 1) the patchy nature of myocardial infiltrates makes sampling error a great concern, 2) the lack of consistent interpretation of EMB samples, even among most experienced pathologists.

The issue of sampling error has been addressed by many authors. Chow and Hauck published on postmortem EMB showing that one sample had a sensibility of 25% to detect myocarditis, and that 5 samples were needed to raise this figure to 66% [17, 18]. Similar experience has been published with the use of EMB to detect allograft rejection [19, 20].

On the other hand, the lack of interobserver agreement in the interpretation of histological samples shows that that the Dallas criteria did not achieve completely their goal. It is remarkable that of the 111 patients enrolled in the Myocarditis Treatment Trial (positive EMB according to Dallas criteria required as inclusion condition) only 64% had the diagnosis confirmed by the expert pathologist panel [21]. In another study where 7 expert pathologists examined the EMB of 16 patients with dilated cardiomyopathy (DCM), interpretation of samples varied remarkably. Diagnosis of myocarditis was made in 11 patients at least by 1 pathologist. But only in 3 patients, three pathologists agreed in the diagnosis, and in 5, two pathologists agreed, showing that even for expert pathologists, interpretation of EMB is quite variable [22].

Some investigators showed that many patients with a clinical presentation suggestive of myocarditis were negative for Dallas criteria but had a PCR positive for viral genomes in the EMB. Martin el al. studied 34 children with clinical presentation suggestive of myocarditis. Twenty-six of the 34 samples were positive for viral genomes but only 13 of the 26 were positive for Dallas criteria [23]. Pauschinger et al. found that 24 of 94 patients with idiopathic dilated cardiomyopathy (DCM), all of them negative for Dallas criteria, were positive for viral genomes [24]. In another study, Pauschinger et al. demonstrated positive PCR for enteroviruses in 45 patients with idiopathic DCM; only 6 were positive for Dallas criteria [25]. Why et al. showed in 120 patients with DCM that 41 were positive for enterovirus genomes in their EMB, but only 5 were positive for Dallas criteria [26].

Dallas criteria also lack prognostic value. Grogan et al. compared the clinical outcome in 27 patients with myocarditis and 58 patients with idiopathic DMC; presence of myocarditis did not affect prognosis [4]. Angelini et al. followed 42 patients with biopsy proven myocarditis, 26 with active myocarditis and 16 with borderline myocarditis also according to Dallas criteria. Heart failure was more frequent in the borderline myocarditis (BM) group than in the acute myocarditis (AM) group. They concluded that myocyte necrosis does not carry prognostic value [5]. Caforio et al. studied 174 patients, with active myocarditis (n=85) or borderline myocarditis (n=89). They concluded that IHC enhanced EMB sensitivity for the diagnosis of myocarditis and that Dallas criteria lacked prognostic value [6]. Kindermann et al. followed 181 patients with clinically suspected myocarditis in whom EMB was performed. Dallas criteria were positive only in 69 patients (38%), but sensitivity was increased bythe use of IHC, which showed inflammation in 91 patients. Dallas criteria also proved of no prognostic value in that study [7].

Moreover, Dallas criteria did not show predictive value to select patients for immunosuppressant therapy. Clinical trials using immunosuppressant treatment for myocarditis did not show, in general, a better outcome in patients who received treatment compared to those who received placebo, even though, some patients improved markedly their left ventricular function after treatment. Dallas criteria did not predict which patients were to improve [21, 27].

The need of new criteria to make the definite diagnosis has been claimed for many authors, but as shown in the papers cited, the Dallas criteria supported by immunohistochemistry remain, at present the "gold standard" for the diagnosis of myocarditis.

5.2. The role of immunohistochemistry

The main problem with the histopathological diagnosis of myocarditis in routine samples is the differentiation between interstitial lymphocytes and other types of cells, mainly fibroblasts and histiocytes.

Schnitt et al. published a pioneer work in 50 consecutive EMBs assessed by two independent observers [28].The use of an immunoperoxidase technique to stain specifically leucocyte common antigen (CLA, now CD45A) had a better interobserver concordance (r=0.83) than hematoxylin – eosin (H&E) samples (r=0.63) in identifying lymphocytes. Intraobserver concordance between IHC and H&E-identified lymphocytes was poor (r=0.28 and r=0.14 respectively). The main drawback of CLA antibodies is that it also stains mast cells and histiocytes. They did not study the impact of the technique in the diagnosis of myocarditis [28].

One of us (JM) emphasized in a pioneer paper in 1990, the need of immunohistochemical staining of lymphocytes for the reliable diagnosis of myocarditis in EMB. The diagnosis of myocarditis was established in 27 patients according to routine staining of EMB samples. We analyzed those samples using antibodies to CLA, κ and λ immunoglobulin light chains and T cell receptor (TCR). Only 14 out of the 27 biopsies showed to have true myocarditis [8]. The technique proved to be useful for diagnosis of myocarditis as a cause of sudden death (figure 9) [30].

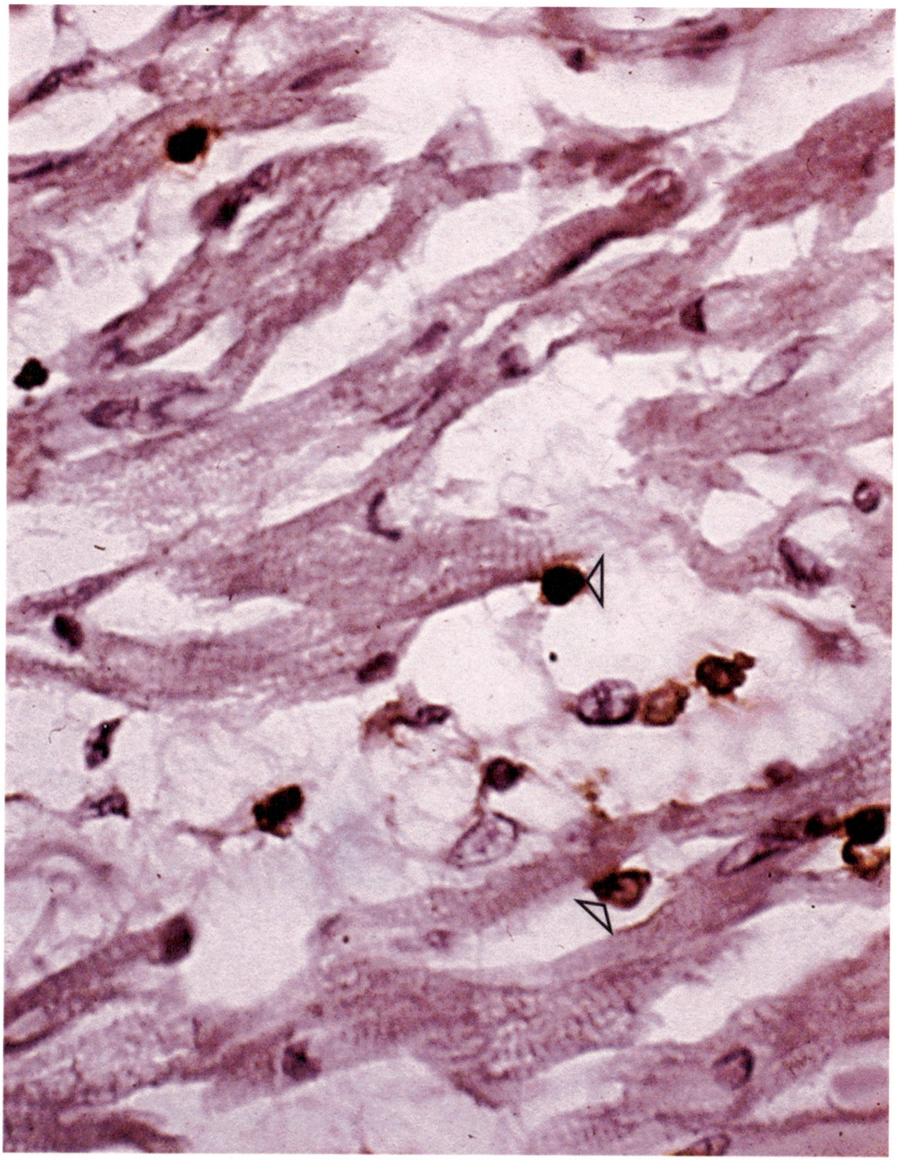

Figure 9. Diffuse myocarditis in a 6 year-old boy found underwater in a swimming pool. There are extensive myocardial injury and marked interstitial edema and apposition of T- lymphocytes to the sarcolemma of necrotic myocytes. Immunoperoxidase for T- lymphocytes. Note the classic picnotic nuclei and cytoplasmic positivity (arrows) X200 [30].

After these papers, new markers and new antibodies have been developed and IHC diagnosis has become more sophisticated. Kühl et al. studied the biopsies of 170 patients with DCM with no history of previous viral disease. EMB were performed and processed for H&E to determine the presence of myocarditis according to Dallas criteria, and for immunohistochemistry using antibodies to CD45RA, CD2, CD3, CD4, CD8, CD45R0 and HLA class I. Only 5% of samples were positive for Dallas criteria, but 48% showed positive staining for one or more of the antibodies, showing a very higher sensitivity of immunohistochemistry to show inflammatory changes in DCM [29].

Feeley et al. showed that antibodies anti CD45R0 were very accurate for the diagnosis of myocardial inflammation in a series of 163 routine autopsies in a general hospital. The only 5 samples that showed more than 14 CD45R0 positive cells per high power field belonged to transplanted patients, of whom three with cardiac rejection and one with a linfoproliferative disorder [30]. Although not designed to study myocarditis, Krous et al. showed that staining with anti CD3 (T lymphocytes) and CD68 (macrophages) was useful to differentiate myocarditis from sudden infant death syndrome and suffocation in EMB of children [31]. And as previously reported, in our hands immunohistochemical staining allowed the diagnosis of unapparent myocarditis as a cause of sudden death in children [32].

In a paper by Caforio et al. immunohistochemistry has been used to reinforce Dallas criteria. More than half of borderline myocarditis diagnosis would have been missed with H&E alone [6]. In this connection, also Kindermann et al showed in their study that only 69 (38%) out of 181 EMB samples were positive for Dallas criteria while 91 (50%) were positive using CD3, CD68 and HLA class II antibodies [7].

5.3. The role of polymerase chain reaction

In the early 1990s many authors published series of cases showing the isolation of different viral genomes with PCR [33-37], but these papers were mainly descriptive of the presence of certain types of viruses in EMB samples and did not assess prognostic or therapeutic value of these findings. However, almost a decade after PCR also proved to be of prognostic value [36]. Frustaci et al. treated 41 patients with biopsy proven myocarditis who presented with ongoing heart failure with complete standard immunosuppressant treatment. Viral genomes were present in biopsy specimens of 17 non responders (85%), including enterovirus (n=5), Epstein-Barr virus (n=5) adenovirus (n=4), both adenovirus and enterovirus (n=1), influenza A virus (n=1), parvovirus-B19 (n=1), and in 3 responders, who were all positive for hepatitis C virus. Cardiac autoantibodies were present in 19 responders (90%) and in none of the nonresponders. The presence of viral genomes was independently associated with failure of immunosuppression to improve ventricular function [38]. Conversely, Camargo et al. demonstrated that children with chronic myocarditis have a favorable response to immunosupressant therapy independently of the presence or not of viral genomes in EMB [39].

Kytö et al. showed in a retrospective analysis of autopsies of 40 fatal myocarditis that viral nucleic acids were found in the hearts of 17 patients (43%), including CMV (15 patients), parvovirus B19 (4 patients), enterovirus (1 patient), and human herpes virus 6 (1 patient). In 4 patients, CMV DNA was found in addition to parvovirus B19 or enterovirus genomes. No adenoviruses, rhinoviruses, or influenza viruses were detected in that study of fatal myocarditis. In 67% of the patients in whom PCR was positive for CMV, *in situ* hybridization revealed viral DNA in cardiomyocytes. Only 1 of these patients was immunocompromised. From these findings it can be concluded that the finding of CMV genome in EMB biopsies of patients with myocarditis carries a particularly bad prognosis [40].

Wilmot et al. also demonstrated the prognostic value of PCR in fulminant myocarditis in 16 children treated with mechanical circulatory support. PCR results were available from 15 patients and were positive in 11. Viral presence was associated with death or need for transplantation (P = 0.011). Upon histological analysis, absence of viral infection and lack of myocardial inflammation were associated with recovery (P values 0.011 and 0.044, respectively) [41].

Mavrogeni et al. followed a cohort of 85 patients with myocarditis. In 71 patients CRM was positive and in 50 EMB was performed. Chlamydia, herpes virus and parvovirus B19 were present in 80 % of EMB samples. In 7 patients with clinical deterioration 1 year after, EMB showed persistence of infectious agent genomes [42].

Viral myocarditis is a known cause of sudden death. In this connection, PCR has been performed in post-mortem samples of patients with sudden death. The test proved to be of diagnostic usefulness in some cases [43, 44].

6. Endomyocardial biopsy as a research tool

The role of EMB as a research tool cannot be undervalued. Almost all papers cited in this chapter have been conducted on EMB samples. Many developments relative to heart disease are due to basic science investigations using EMB. In this regard, many advances in the understanding of genetic expression in the failing heart have been made thanks to the possibility of obtaining heart muscle samples [45-48].

In the specific field of myocarditis, EMB will surely allow to identify better predictors of mortality, need of transplantation and response to certain drugs or therapeutic strategies by the discover of new molecular markers of inflammation, tissue damage or survival. With PCR the prognostic value of viral genome presence will be better defined promptly and, in the future, the expression of certain myocyte genes will surely introduce a new tool to predict outcomes.

7. Conclusions

As shown by the data revised here, EMB is an important diagnostic tool in myocarditis. It still remains the gold standard for the definite diagnosis. Dallas criteria, although severely questioned by many authors, still remain a reference method to establish diagnosis and are generally required as inclusion criteria in clinical investigation. On the other hand, it helps distinguishing lymphocytic myocarditis from other entities, like giant cell myocarditis, necrotizing eosinophilic myocarditis or sarcoidosis, which may guide treatment and prognosis.

The introduction of IHC and PCR provided new tools for evaluating EMB samples. Although not yet standardized adequately, they have shown to give valuable prognostic and therapeutic information. They have become routine testing in myocarditis.

Author details

Julián González[1], Francisco Salgado[1], Francisco Azzato[1], Giuseppe Ambrosio[2] and Jose Milei[1]

1 Instituto de Investigaciones Cardiológicas Prof. A. Taquini – UBA – CONICET, Facultad de Medicina, Universidad de Buenos Aires, Argentina

2 University of Perugia School of Medicine, Perugia, Italy

References

[1] Ferrans VJ, Roberts WC. Myocardial biopsy: a useful diagnostic procedure or only a research tool? Am J Cardiol. 1978 May 1;41(5):965-7.

[2] Cooper LT, Baughman KL, Feldman AM, Frustaci A, Jessup M, Kuhl U, et al. The Role of Endomyocardial Biopsy in the Management of Cardiovascular Disease. Circulation. 2007 November 6, 2007;116(19):2216-33.

[3] Aretz H, Billingham M, Edwards W, Factor S, Fallon J, Fenoglio JJ, et al. Myocarditis: a histopathologic definition and classification. American Journal of Cardiovascular Pathology. 1987;1(1):3 - 14.

[4] Grogan M, Redfield MM, Bailey KR, Reeder GS, Gersh BJ, Edwards WD, et al. Long-term outcome of patients with biopsy-proved myocarditis: Comparison with idiopathic dilated cardiomyopathy. Journal of the American College of Cardiology. 1995;26(1): 80-4.

[5] Angelini A, Crosato M, Boffa GM, Calabrese F, Calzolari V, Chioin R, et al. Active versus borderline myocarditis: clinicopathological correlates and prognostic implications. Heart. 2002 March 1, 2002;87(3):210-5.

[6] Caforio ALP, Calabrese F, Angelini A, Tona F, Vinci A, Bottaro S, et al. A prospective study of biopsy-proven myocarditis: prognostic relevance of clinical and aetiopathogenetic features at diagnosis. European Heart Journal. 2007 June 1, 2007;28(11):1326-33.

[7] Kindermann I, Kindermann M, Kandolf R, Klingel K, Bültmann B, Müller T, et al. Predictors of Outcome in Patients With Suspected Myocarditis. Circulation. 2008 August 5, 2008;118(6):639-48.

[8] Milei J, Bortman G, Fernández-Alonso G, Grancelli H, Beigelman R. Immunohistochemical Staining of Lymphocytes for the Reliable Diagnosis of Myocarditis in Endomyocardial Biopsies. Cardiology. 1990;77(2):77-85.

[9] Report of the 1995 World Health Organization/International Society and Federation of Cardiology Task Force on the Definition and Classification of Cardiomyopathies. Circulation. 1996 March 1, 1996;93(5):841-2.

[10] Blauwet LA, Cooper LT. Myocarditis. Prog Cardiovasc Dis. 2010 Jan-Feb;52(4):274-88.

[11] Cunningham KS, Veinot JP, Butany J. An approach to endomyocardial biopsy interpretation. Journal of Clinical Pathology. 2006 February 1, 2006;59(2):121-9.

[12] Sakakibara S, Konno S. Endomyocardial Biopsy. Japanese Heart Journal. 1962;3(6): 537-43.

[13] Takemura G, Fujiwara H, Horike K, Mukoyama M, Saito Y, Nakao K, et al. Ventricular expression of atrial natriuretic polypeptide and its relations with hemodynamics and histology in dilated human hearts. Immunohistochemical study of the endomyocardial biopsy specimens. Circulation. 1989 November 1, 1989;80(5):1137-47.

[14] Billingham M. Pathology of Heart Transplantantion. In: Solez K, Racusen L, Billingham M, editors. Solid Organ Transplant Rejection: mechanisms, pathology and diagnosis. New York: Marcel Dekker, Inc.; 1996. p. 137 - 59.

[15] Deckers JW, Hare JM, Baughman KL. Complications of transvenous right ventricular endomyocardial biopsy in adult patients with cardiomyopathy: A seven-year survey of 546 consecutive diagnostic procedures in a tertiary referral center. Journal of the American College of Cardiology. 1992;19(1):43-7.

[16] Baughman KL. Diagnosis of Myocarditis. Circulation. 2006 January 31, 2006;113(4): 593-5.

[17] Chow LH, Radio SJ, Sears TD, McManus BM. Insensitivity of right ventricular endomyocardial biopsy in the diagnosis of myocarditis. Journal of the American College of Cardiology. 1989;14(4):915-20.

[18] Hauck A, Kearney D, Edwards W. Evaluation of postmortem endomyocardial biopsy specimens from 38 patients with lymphocytic myocarditis: implications for role of sampling error. Mayo Clinic Proceedings. 1989;64:1235 - 45.

[19] Spiegelhalter DJ, Stovin PGI. An analysis of repeated biopsies following cardiac transplantation. Statistics in Medicine. 1983;2(1):33-40.

[20] Zerbe T, Arena V. Diagnostic reliability of endomyocardial biopsy for assessment of cardiac allograft rejection. Human Pathology. 1988;19:1307 - 14.

[21] Mason JW, O'Connell JB, Herskowitz A, Rose NR, McManus BM, Billingham ME, et al. A Clinical Trial of Immunosuppressive Therapy for Myocarditis. New England Journal of Medicine. 1995;333(5):269-75.

[22] Shanes JG, Ghali J, Billingham ME, Ferrans VJ, Fenoglio JJ, Edwards WD, et al. Interobserver variability in the pathologic interpretation of endomyocardial biopsy results. Circulation. 1987 February 1, 1987;75(2):401-5.

[23] Martin AB, Webber S, Fricker FJ, Jaffe R, Demmler G, Kearney D, et al. Acute myocarditis. Rapid diagnosis by PCR in children. Circulation. 1994 July 1, 1994;90(1):330-9.

[24] Pauschinger M, Bowles NE, Fuentes-Garcia FJ, Pham V, Kühl U, Schwimmbeck PL, et al. Detection of Adenoviral Genome in the Myocardium of Adult Patients With Idiopathic Left Ventricular Dysfunction. Circulation. 1999 March 16, 1999;99(10):1348-54.

[25] Pauschinger M, Doerner A, Kuehl U, Schwimmbeck PL, Poller W, Kandolf R, et al. Enteroviral RNA Replication in the Myocardium of Patients With Left Ventricular Dysfunction and Clinically Suspected Myocarditis. Circulation. 1999 February 23, 1999;99(7):889-95.

[26] Why HJ, Meany BT, Richardson PJ, Olsen EG, Bowles NE, Cunningham L, et al. Clinical and prognostic significance of detection of enteroviral RNA in the myocardium of patients with myocarditis or dilated cardiomyopathy. Circulation. 1994 June 1, 1994;89(6):2582-9.

[27] McNamara DM, Holubkov R, Starling RC, Dec GW, Loh E, Torre-Amione G, et al. Controlled Trial of Intravenous Immune Globulin in Recent-Onset Dilated Cardiomyopathy. Circulation. 2001 May 8, 2001;103(18):2254-9.

[28] Schnitt S, Ciano P, Schoen F. Quantitation of Lymphocytes in Endomyocardial Biopsies: Use and Limitations of Antibodies to Leucocyte Common Antigen. Human Pathology. 1987;18(8):796 - 800.

[29] Kühl U, Noutsias M, Seeberg B, Schultheiss HP. Immunohistological evidence for a chronic intramyocardial inflammatory process in dilated cardiomyopathy. Heart. 1996 March 1, 1996;75(3):295-300.

[30] Feeley KM, Harris J, Suvarna SK. Necropsy diagnosis of myocarditis: a retrospective study using CD45RO immunohistochemistry. Journal of Clinical Pathology. 2000 February 1, 2000;53(2):147-9.

[31] Krous HF, Ferandos C, Masoumi H, Arnold J, Haas EA, Stanley C, et al. Myocardial Inflammation, Cellular Death, and Viral Detection in Sudden Infant Death Caused by SIDS, Suffocation, or Myocarditis. Pediatr Res. 2009;66(1):17-21.

[32] Forcada P, Beigelman R, Milei J. Inapparent myocarditis and sudden death in pediatrics. Diagnosis by immunohistochemical staining. International Journal of Cardiology. 1996;56(1):93-7.

[33] Jin O, Sole MJ, Butany JW, Chia WK, McLaughlin PR, Liu P, et al. Detection of enterovirus RNA in myocardial biopsies from patients with myocarditis and cardiomyopathy using gene amplification by polymerase chain reaction. Circulation. 1990 July 1, 1990;82(1):8-16.

[34] Koide H, Kitaura Y, Deguchi H, Ukimura A, Kawamura K, Hirai K. Genomic Detection of Enteroviruses in The Myocardium : Studies on animal hearts with coxsackievirus B3 myocarditis and endomyocardial biopsies from patients with myocarditis and dilated cardiomyopathy: Molecular Analysis of the Pathophysiology of Cardiomypathy. Japanese Circulation Journal. 1992;56(10):1081-93.

[35] Hilton DA, Variend S, Pringle JH. Demonstration of coxsackie virus RNA in formalin-fixed tissue sections from childhood myocarditis cases by in situ hybridization and the polymerase chain reaction. The Journal of Pathology. 1993;170(1):45-51.

[36] Nichlson F, Ajetunmobi J, Li M, Shackleton E, Starket W, Illavia S, et al. Molecular detection and serotypic analysis of enterovirus RNA in archival specimens from patients with acute myocarditis. British Heart Journal. 1995;74(5):522 - 7.

[37] Fujioka S, Koide H, Kitaura Y, Deguchi H, Kawamura K, Hirai K. Molecular detection and differentiation of enteroviruses in endomyocardial biopsies and pericardial effusions from dilated cardiomyopathy and myocarditis. American Heart Journal 1996;131(4):760-5.

[38] Frustaci A, Chimenti C, Calabrese F, Pieroni M, Thiene G, Maseri A. Immunosuppressive Therapy for Active Lymphocytic Myocarditis. Circulation. 2003 February 18, 2003;107(6):857-63.

[39] Camargo PR, Okay TS, Yamamoto L, Del Negro GMB, Lopes AA. Myocarditis in children and detection of viruses in myocardial tissue: Implications for immunosuppressive therapy. International Journal of Cardiology. 2011;148(2):204-8.

[40] Kytö V, Vuorinen T, Saukko P, Lautenschlager I, Lignitz E, Saraste A, et al. Cytomegalovirus Infection of the Heart Is Common in Patients with Fatal Myocarditis. Clinical Infectious Diseases. 2005 March 1, 2005;40(5):683-8.

[41] Wilmot I, Morales DLS, Price JF, Rossano JW, Kim JJ, Decker JA, et al. Effectiveness of Mechanical Circulatory Support in Children With Acute Fulminant and Persistent Myocarditis. Journal of Cardiac Failure. 2011;17(6):487-94.

[42] Mavrogeni S, Spargias C, Bratis C, Kolovou G, Markussis V, Papadopoulou E, et al. Myocarditis as a precipitating factor for heart failure: evaluation and 1-year follow-up using cardiovascular magnetic resonance and endomyocardial biopsy. European Journal of Heart Failure. 2011 August 1, 2011;13(8):830-7.

[43] De Salvia A, De Leo D, Carturan E, Basso C. Sudden cardiac death, borderline myocarditis and molecular diagnosis: evidence or assumption? Medicine, Science and the Law. 2011 October 1, 2011;51(suppl 1):S27-S9.

[44] Gaaloul I, Riabi S, Harrath R, Evans M, H Salem N, Mlayeh S, et al. Sudden unexpected death related to enterovirus myocarditis: histopathology, immunohistochemstry and molecular pathology diagnosis at post-mortem. BMC Infectious Diseases. 2012;12(1): 212.

[45] Feldman AM, Ray PE, Silan CM, Mercer JA, Minobe W, Bristow MR. Selective gene expression in failing human heart. Quantification of steady-state levels of messenger RNA in endomyocardial biopsies using the polymerase chain reaction. Circulation. 1991 June 1, 1991;83(6):1866-72.

[46] Ladenson PW, Sherman SI, Baughman KL, Ray PE, Feldman AM. Reversible alterations in myocardial gene expression in a young man with dilated cardiomyopathy and hypothyroidism. Proceedings of the National Academy of Sciences. 1992 June 15, 1992;89(12):5251-5.

[47] Bristow MR, Minobe WA, Raynolds MV, Port JD, Rasmussen R, Ray PE, et al. Reduced beta 1 receptor messenger RNA abundance in the failing human heart. The Journal of Clinical Investigation. 1993;92(6):2737-45.

[48] Lowes BD, Zolty R, Minobe WA, Robertson AD, Leach S, Hunter L, et al. Serial Gene Expression Profiling in the Intact Human Heart. The Journal of Heart and Lung Transplantation: the official publication of the International Society for Heart Transplantation. 2006;25(5):579-88.

Section 4

Myocarditis in Special Populations

Chapter 5

Pathogenesis of Chronic Chagasic Myocarditis

Julián González, Francisco Azzato,
Giusepe Ambrosio and José Milei

Additional information is available at the end of the chapter

http://dx.doi.org/10.5772/55387

1. Introduction

Chronic chagasic cardiomyopathy (CCC) is the most serious manifestation of the chronic form of Chagas' disease and constitutes the most common type of chronic myocarditis in the world [1-5]. Chagas' disease, a chronic illness caused by the flagellate parasite *Trypanosoma cruzi* (*T. cruzi*), was first described in 1909 by the Brazilian physician Carlos Chagas [6]. The insect vectors of the disease are present throughout most of South and Central America, and their zone of distribution extends across the southern United States [7]. It was estimated by year 2000, that in endemic areas 40 million people were considered to be at risk of infection, being 20 million already infected. Every year near 200,000 new cases are expected to happen, and 21,000 deaths per year occur [8].

Although always considered to be confined to Latin America, due to migratory movements from endemic countries to Europe and North America, Chagas' disease is being detected more frequently in developed countries. Europe is estimated to have from 24,001 to 38,708 (lower or upper limit of estimate, respectively) immigrants with *T. cruzi* infection [1]. In the United States 6 autochthonous cases, five transfusion related cases and five transplant associated cases have been reported, but migratory movements still remain the main source of Chagas' disease. It has been estimated that around 89,221 to 693,302 infected Latin Americans migrated to the United States in the period 1981 to 2005 [3].

Two phases of the disease can be distinguished: (1) acute phase, with transiently high concentration of parasites in tissue and blood, nonspecific symptoms, and a 5% myocarditis incidence, lasting 4 – 8 weeks; and (2) chronic phase, lasting lifelong. Chronic phase can be presented as indeterminate form, characterized by lack of symptoms and normal ECG and normal radiographic examination of the chest, esophagus and colon. Approximately 60 – 70% of patients remain in this form for the rest of their lives. Only 20 - 40% of infected individuals,

10 - 30 years after the original acute infection, will develop cardiac, digestive or mixed form of the disease, characterized by the appearance of megavicera (dilated cardiomyopathy, megaesophagus and/or megacolon). It poses a substantial public health burden due to high morbidity and mortality [3, 7, 9].

CCC is manifested by a chronic, diffuse, progressive fibrosing myocarditis that involves not only the working myocardium but also the atrioventricular (AV) conduction system, autonomic nervous system and microcirculation [10 - 12]. This leads to cardiomegaly, cardiac failure, arrhythmias, thromboembolism, and death [11]. Colon and esophagus are also commonly affected by Chagas' disease, being megacolon with constipation and megaesofagus with achalasia also features of the disease [7].

2. Pathogenesis of Chagas' myocarditis

Milei et al. proposed a combined theory that could explain the pathogenic mechanism in chronic chagasic myocarditis [2, 13] that has been previously reviewed by us [14]. This hypothesis is based on three ingredients: the parasite, host immune system and fibrosis. These ingredients are proposed as being the primary causative agents of damage on myocardial tissue, conduction system, autonomic ganglia and nerves and microvasculature.

2.1. First ingredient: The parasite

The role of *T. cruzi* in the chronic phase has been previously underestimated due to the fact that its presence was believed to be scarce and unrelated to the inflammatory infiltrate present at this stage. Nowadays, the involvement of the parasite in the chronic phase has been well documented. Using dissimilar methods, different authors demonstrated either the persistence of *T. cruzi* or parasite antigens in mice [15], the parasite DNA sequence amplified by the polymerase chain reaction (PCR) [16, 17], *T. cruzi* antigens from inflammatory lesions in human chagasic cardiomyopathy [18], or the immunohistochemical finding of the parasite in endomyocardial biopsies with PCR confirmation [19]. This would suggest a direct role for the parasite in the perpetuation of myocardial inflammation. In other words, the antigen stimulation would persist throughout the chronic stage, even though the parasites are not morphologically detectable by light microscopy [20].

The role of parasitemia is more controversial. High parasitemia correlated with severity of disease in one report [21], but showed no association in another [22]. Interestingly, it has been observed that immunosuppression reactivates rather than ameliorates the disease, as seen in patients receiving immunosuppressive therapy to prevent transplant rejection and in AIDS patients. Accordingly, many experimental models where strains of genetically manipulated mice lacking various immune functions showed increased susceptibility to develop the disease [23].

2.1.1. Life cycle of Trypanosoma cruzi (Figure 1)

When a reduviid bug feeds from an infected mammal, it takes up circulating trypomastigotes, which reach then the bug's gut. There, they differentiate to amastigotes, which proliferate and start to differentiate into epimastigotes. In this process, when amastigote is still sphere-shaped but has developed its flagellum, some authors call this stage spheromastigotes. Then, it elongates its cell body and flagellum, taking the classical epimastigote shape. At this stage, the parasite undergoes metacyclogenesis, differentiating in metacyclic trypomastigotes, the infective form for mammals. When the bug feeds again, it excretes trypomastigotes with feces, which in turn reach blood torrent through bug's wound. Trypomastigotes can infect a wide variety of host cells, within them it differentiate into amastigotes and proliferate. Then, they can differentiate into trypomastigotes again, reach circulation and infect new cells. If an uninfected bug feeds from the animal in the moment of parasitemia, cycle starts again [24].

2.1.2. Genetic variability of Trypanosoma cruzi and its relation to its pathogenesis

The genetics of *T. cruzi* caught the attention of researchers in late 80' and early 90'. First studies on variability were performed analyzing electrophoretic variants on cellular enzymes. The

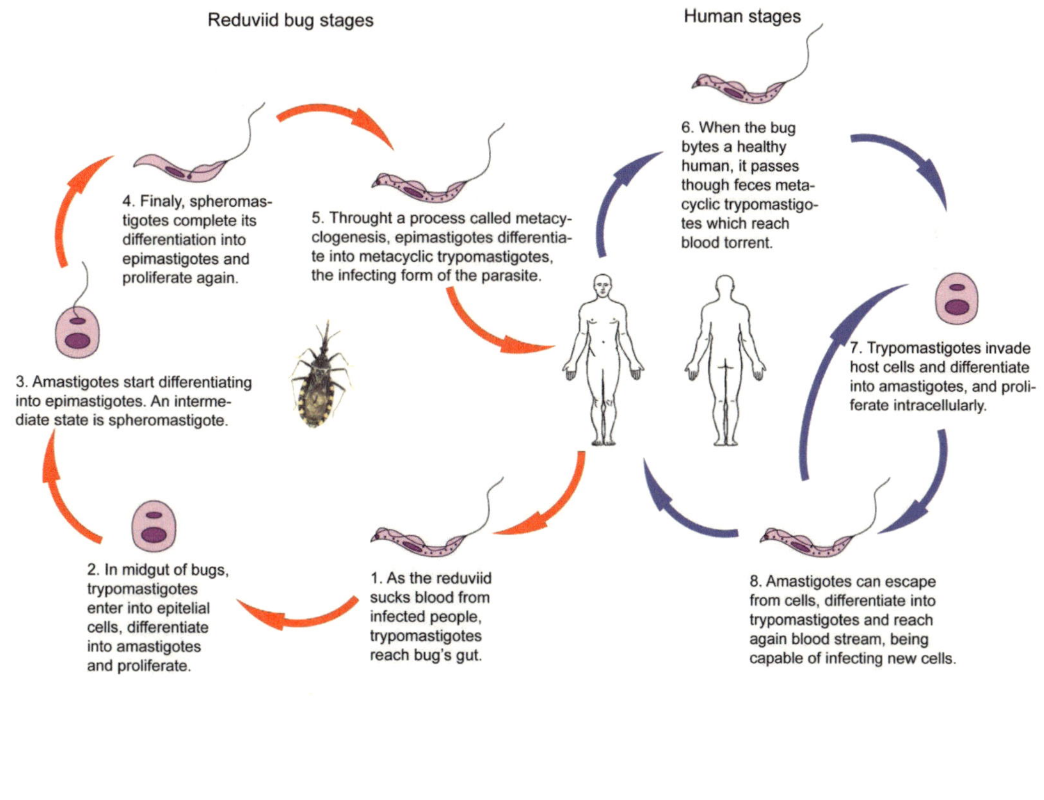

Figure 1. Life cycle of Trypanosoma cruzi

groups resulting were called zymodemes and were named Z1, Z2, Z3. Only Z2 was associated with domestic transmission cycle.

THe development of PCR based techniques allowed the study of new variant regions and the characterization of multiple variants of a great number of genes. All these variants showed significant correlation with each other, suggesting the existence of two subtypes of *T. Cruzi* based on these data [25]. Moreover, *T. cruzi II* which is clearly linked to human pathology, being *T. cruzi I* mainly related to infection of wild sylvatic mammals. Even, applying LSSP-PCR to the study of the variable region of kinetoplast minicircle from T. cruzi provided evidence of a differential tissue distribution of genetically diverse T. cruzi populations in chronic Chagas' disease, suggesting that the genetic variability of the parasite is one of the determining factors of the clinical form of the disease [26].

2.1.3. Cell host invasion and intracellular survival by Trypanosoma cruzi

Once *T. cruzi* reaches blood torrent, it invades a great variety of cells in the host. When parasiting non phagocytic cells, *T. cruzi* uses some surface glycoproteins to attach to cell: gp82, gp30 and gp35/50. All three glycoproteins are known to induce calcium mobilization from intracellular reservoirs. Gp82 is linked to the phospholipase C (PLC) and inositol 1,4,5 – triphosphate (IP3). Gp 35/50is associated to increasing intracellular levels of cyclic AMP. On the other side, cruzipain, a protein known to be secreted by *T. cruzi*, acts on kininogen and produces bradykinin, which binds to its receptor, further increasing intracellular calcium. Increased intracellular calcium produces modifications in cytoskeleton that lead to parasite endocytosis [27].

In the parasitoforous vacuole, mainly by the action of gp85/TS a glycoprotein with trans-sialidase action, and TcTox, a protease, the parasite degrades the membrane of the vacuole, escapes from it and proliferates within the cell [28].

2.1.4. Molecular mimicry

The induction of autoimmunity by similarities between *T. cruzi* and host epitopes has been long proposed as a mechanism that leads to tissue damage in the chronic phase of the disease. Both humoral and cellular autoimmune responses have been described, but we will discuss them in more detail in the section of immune system. The real importance of molecular mimicry in the pathogenesis of chagasic myocarditis is still a matter of debate [29].

Although it seems that in some cases this mechanism triggers autoimmunity, in many others, autoimmunity seems to be an epiphenomenon of cellular destruction, with exposition of intracellular epitopes not normally exposed to the immune system. This, in turn may activate autoreactive lymphocytes leading to the appearance of autoantibodies that are not the cause of damage, rather a consequence [29].

The most important cross reacting epitopes of *T. cruzi* and the correspondent epitopes in humans are listed in table 1, as well as the kind of immune response they elicit.

http://dx.doi.org/10.5772/55387

2.2. Second ingredient: Host immune system

When the three ingredients theory was first proposed [2, 13], second ingredients were mainly T lymphocytes and macrophages. In the subsequent years some evidence grew about the participation of humoral immune system through autoantibodies in the pathogenesis. As a consequence, the whole immune system of the host is now considered as the second ingredient.

As described earlier, mononuclear cells persist in the chronic stage of the disease, contributing to the inflammation through its products of secretion or through its own cytotoxicity (suppressor T cells) and cytolytic action (macrophages) [13]. As previously stated, molecular mimicry may be the main explanation of autoimmunity, triggering both cellular and humoral autoreactivity [29]. Figure 2 summarizes the most important immune events in CCC pathogenesis.

Parasite antigen	Human Antigen	Immune reaction
B13	Cardiac myosin heavy chain	Autoantibodies Autoreactive T cells
R13 (ribosomal protein)	Ribosomal protein β_1-adrenergic receptor M_2-muscarinic receptor 38-kDa heart antigen	Autoantibodies
Ribosomal protein PO	β_1-adrenergic receptor	Autoantibodies
FL-160	47-kDA neuron protein	Autoantibodies
Shed acute-phase antigen (SAPA)	Cha antigen	Autoreactive T cells
TENU2845/36 kDa	Cha antigen	Autoantibodies
Calcireticulin	Calcireticulin	Autoantibodies Autoreactive T cells
Galactosyl-cerebrosides	Galactosyl-cerebrosides	Autoantibodies
Unknown	Neurons, liver, kidney, testis	Autoantibodies
Sulphated glycolipids	Neurons	Autoantibodies
150-kDa protein	Smooth and striated muscle	Autoantibodies
Cruzipain	Cardiac myosin heavy chain M_2-muscarinic receptor	Autoantibodies
Microsomal fraction	Heart and skeletal muscle	Autoantibodies
Cytoskeleton	95-kDa myosin tail	Autoantibodies
SRA	Skeletal muscle Ca^{2+} dependent SRA	Autoantibodies
MAP	MAP (brain)	Autoantibodies
Soluble extract	Myelin basic protein	Autoantibodies Autoreactive T cells
55-kDa membrane protein	28-kDa Lymphocyte membrane protein	Autoantibodies

Table 1. Examples of cross-reacting epitopes [12, 29]

A

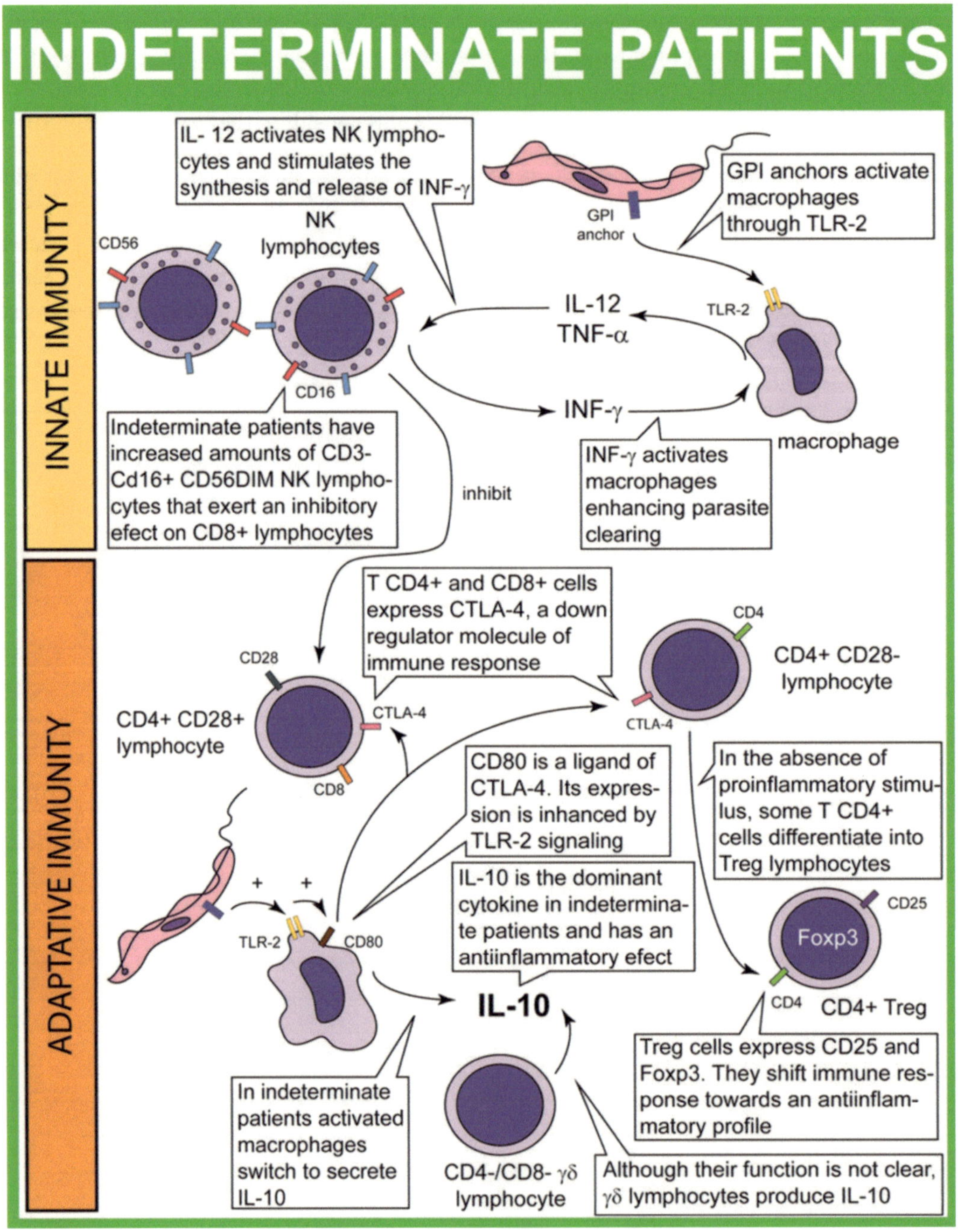
INDETERMINATE PATIENTS
INNATE IMMUNITY
IL- 12 activates NK lymphocytes and stimulates the synthesis and release of INF-γ
GPI anchors activate macrophages through TLR-2
GPI anchor
CD56
NK lymphocytes
IL-12
TNF-α
TLR-2
CD16
INF-γ
macrophage
Indeterminate patients have increased amounts of CD3-Cd16+ CD56DIM NK lymphocytes that exert an inhibitory efect on CD8+ lymphocytes
inhibit
INF-γ activates macrophages enhancing parasite clearing
ADAPTATIVE IMMUNITY
T CD4+ and CD8+ cells express CTLA-4, a down regulator molecule of immune response
CD4
CD4+ CD28- lymphocyte
CD28
CD4+ CD28+ lymphocyte
CTLA-4
CTLA-4
CD8
CD80 is a ligand of CTLA-4. Its expression is inhanced by TLR-2 signaling
In the absence of proinflammatory stimulus, some T CD4+ cells differentiate into Treg lymphocytes
IL-10 is the dominant cytokine in indeterminate patients and has an antiinflammatory efect
+
+
TLR-2
CD80
CD25
Foxp3
IL-10
CD4
CD4+ Treg
Treg cells express CD25 and Foxp3. They shift immune response towards an antiinflammatory profile
In indeterminate patients activated macrophages switch to secrete IL-10
CD4-/CD8- γδ lymphocyte
Although their function is not clear, γδ lymphocytes produce IL-10

http://dx.doi.org/10.5772/55387

B

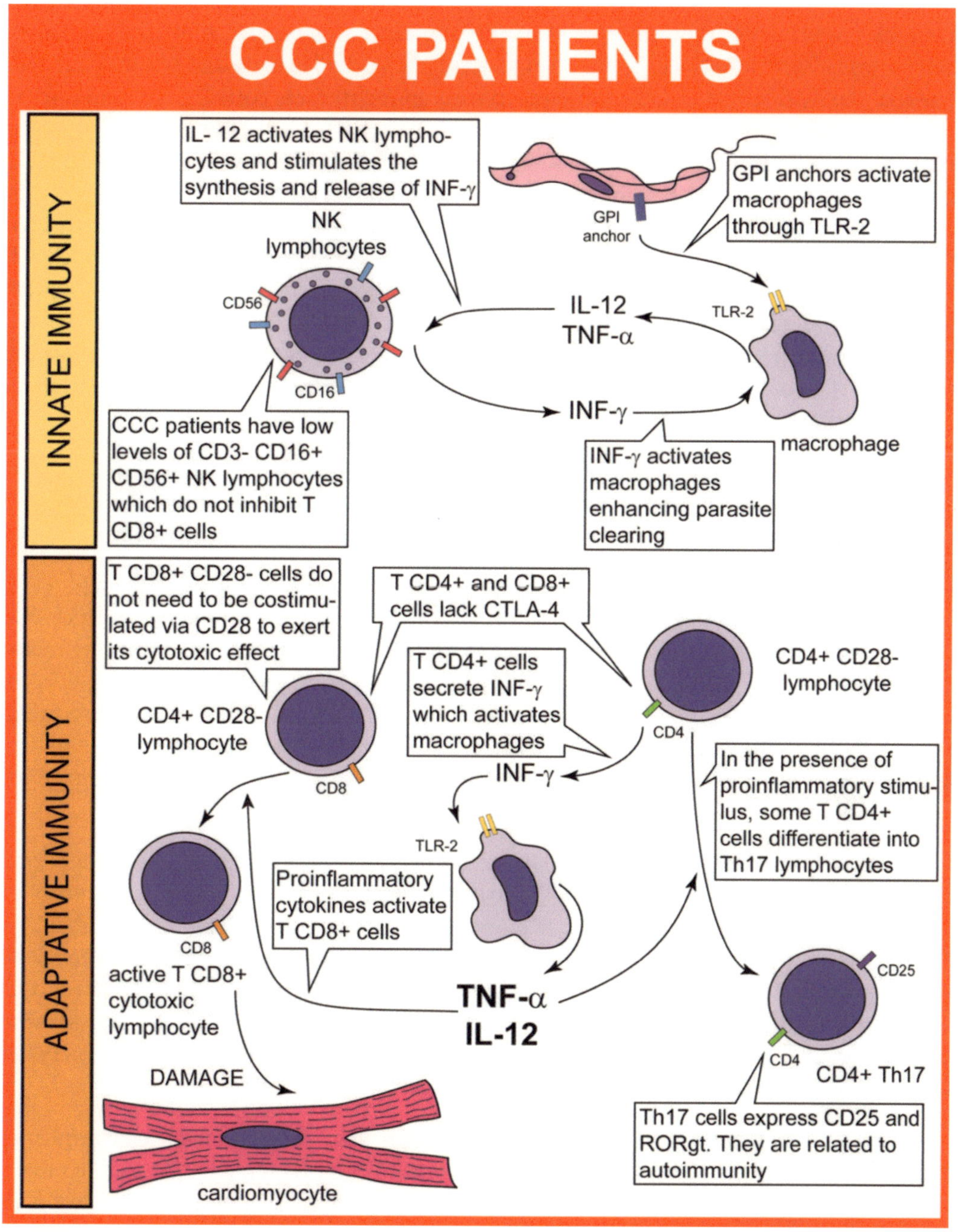

Figure 2. A. The immune pathogenesis of Chagas disease in indeterminate patients. The presence on numerous down regulating mechanisms shift the response towards an anti-inflammatory profile. B. The immune pathogenesis of Chagas disease in CCC patients. Cells evolve towards a proinflammatory profile, with development of autoimmunity.

2.2.1. Innate immunity

In recent years innate immunity came to the attention of researchers of Chagas' disease pathogenesis. The role of NK cells has been particularly studied in early and late indeterminate phases of the disease and in CCC patients. In early indeterminate patients, compared to non infected people, increased values of pre-natural killer (NK)-cells ($CD3^-$ $CD16^+$ $CD56^-$), and higher values of proinflammatory monocytes ($CD14^+$ $CD16^+$ HLA-DR^{++}) were found. The higher values of activated B lymphocytes ($CD19^+$ $CD23^+$) contrasted with impaired T cell activation, indicated by lower values of $CD4^+$ $CD38^+$ and $CD4^+$ HLA-DR^+ lymphocytes, a lower frequency of $CD8^+$ $CD38^+$ and $CD8^+$ HLA-DR^+ cells; a decreased frequency of $CD4^+$ $CD25^{HIGH}$ regulatory T cells was also observed. All these data suggest a rather proinflammatory profile [30]. This profile may be useful to limit parasitemia and confine infection to tissues. In fact, it has been demonstrated that NK cells are important in defence against the spread of parasitic infection [31], and are an important source of INF-γ, a key cytokine to activate macrophages and help with parasite clearance [32].

In late indeterminate phase, $CD3^-CD16^+CD56^+$ and $CD3^-CD16^+CD56^{DIM}$ NK cells are increased but are in normal range in CCC patients, suggesting a protective role for them [33]. NK cells showing $CD56^{DIM}$ may play a role in the down modulation of cytotoxic deleterious T $CD8^+$ response reported in CCC patients [34].

Monocytes display different cytokine profile. In indeterminate patients they produce more IL-10 [35] while in CCC patients they produce more TNF-α [36], leading to a proinflammatory profile that could be responsible for chronic myocarditis. Conversely *in vitro* experiments culturing moncytes from indeterminate and CCC patients showed a predominant production of INF-γ in the former and IL-10 in the later [37]. Also, monocytes of indeterminate patients showed downregulation of Fc-γR, TLR and CR1 molecules, related to an impaired phagocytic capacity [38].

Toll-like receptors (TLR) are also implied in the response to acute infection with *T. cruzi*. TLR-2 has been shown to recognize GPI surface molecules from the parasite. In vitro and in vivo studies have demonstrated that macrofages stimulated with GPIs through TLR-2/CD14 receptors produce NO, TNF-α and IL-12 [39]. Toll-like receptor 4 (TLR4)-deficiency genotype D299G/T399I occurred more frequently in asymptomatic (14.8%) than CCC patients. TLR1-I602S, TLR2-R753Q, TLR6-S249P, and MAL/TIRAP-S180L did not associate with CD or CCC. These findings indicate that curbed TLR4 activation might be beneficial in preventing CCC [40].

A key role of complement in infection control has been clearly established. The complement activating molecules C1q, C3, mannan-binding lectin and ficolins bound to all strains analysed; however, C3b and C4b deposition assays revealed that T. cruzi activates mainly the lectin and alternative complement pathways in non-immune human serum [41]. Mannose-binding lectin (MBL) initiates complement on *Trypanosoma cruzi* through the MBL-associated serine protease 2 (MASP2). MASP2 polymorphisms, specialy g.1961795C, p.371D diplotype (short CD), occurred at a higher frequency among symptomatic patients, compared with the indeterminate group, highlighting the importance of complement in the pathogenesis of CCC [42].

2.2.2. Cellular adaptative immunity

The role of immune cells in the pathogenesis of Chagas' heart disease has been de dominant hypothesis for many years. The paucity of parasite cells in the inflamed myocardium and the presence throughout the evolution of the disease of macrophages and lymphocytes in patched infiltrates lead to this hypotesis. As early as in 1929, Magariños Torres, observing those infiltrates postulated an "allergic" mechanism for CCC. Further, Mazza and Jörg followed this thought and supported the "allergic" theory [13].

The study of circulating lymphocytes in peripheral blood of chagasic patients showed an increase in the percentages and actual numbers of double-positive cells of the phenotype CD3+/HLA-DR+, as well as decrease in the percentage of CD45RA+/CD4+ and CD45RA+/CD8+ T cells, indicating greater numbers of activated T cells circulating. Consistent parallel increases were seen also in the B lymphocyte subset which stained double-positive for CD19/CD5 [43]. These results were similar for both indeterminate and CCC patients. Moreover, T cells from chagasic patients do not express the co-stimulatory molecule CD28 [44] but express high levels of HLA-DR molecules [45]. Some interesting differences were demonstrated between indeterminate and CCC patients. $CD28^-$ T cells in indeterminate patients showed expression of CTLA-4, which recognizes the same ligands as CD28, but instead of inducing cell activation it causes down modulation of T cells. On the contrary, T cells in CCC patients do not up-regulate CTLA-4 [46].

Monocytes from indeterminate patients, when infected in vitro with *T. cruzi*, express low levels of HLA-DR and high levels of CD80, a ligand for CTLA-4 [47]. The interaction of these monocytes with $CTLA\text{-}4^+$ T cells leads to the expression of IL-10, a cytokine known to down-modulate inflammatory responses [35]. This is not observed in CCC patients. $CD28^-$ T cells, not expressing CTLA-4, express TNF-α and INF-γ [44].

In the same direction, $CD4^-CD8^-$ $\gamma\delta$ T cells are found to be increased in indeterminate patients compared with CCC ones. These cells are also linked to the production of IL-10 and a down modulatory effect on inflammation [48].

Cells infiltrating myocardium have also been studied. As demonstrated with immunostaining of endomyocardial biopsies by our group, leukocytes infiltrating myocardium in Chagas' disease were approximately 50% macrophages, and 50% lymphocytes, mainly T lymphocytes [49]. Further immunohistochemical characterization of these cells with CD45R for lymphocytes, CD20 and lambda and kappa light chains for B lymphocytes, CD45R0 for T lymphocytes and CD68 for macrophages, confirmed these findings [2].

Autoreactive T cells have caught the attention of many investigators. In experimental models, $CD4^+$ T cells from infected mice showed a proliferative response to the exposition to human cardiac myosin heavy chain and to *T. cruzi* B13 protein. They also arrested the beating of fetal heart cells and, more importantly, induced myocarditis in immunized mice and promoted rejection of transplanted normal hearts in the absence of *T. cruzi* [50]. Also, it has been described that T cells infiltrating the myocardium of chagasic patients cross react with human cardiac myosin heavy chain and to *T. cruzi* B13 protein and express high levels of INF-γ and low levels of IL-4, switching to a Th1 profile [51].

A second group of autoreactive T cells have been characterized, that react to Cha antigen in human heart. Cha antigen is a protein in human myocardium of unknown function that is recognized sera from chagasic patients. When anti-Cha T cells are transferred to non infected mice, they cause myocarditis and stimulate anti-Cha autoantibodies production [52].

In recent years, a newly described T cell, named Treg, has come to attention in relation to Chagas' disease pathogenesis. These cells are characterized by the expression of CD4 and CD25. Treg cells are increased in indeterminate patients compared to CCC, which correlates negatively with levels of activated $CD8^{+}$ [33]. In a recent review on the role of these cells on the pathogenesis of CCC it is highlighted that indeterminate patients have a higher frequency of Treg cells, suggesting that an expansion of those cells could be beneficial, possibly by limiting strong cytotoxic activity and tissue damage. Indeterminate patients also show an activated status of Treg cells based on low expression of CD62L and high expression of CD40L, CD69, and CD54 by cells from all chagasic patients after T. cruzi antigenic stimulation. Moreover, there was an increase in the frequency of the population of $Foxp3^{+}$ $CD25^{High}CD4^{+}$ cells that was also IL-10^{+} in the IND group, whereas in the cardiac (CARD) group, there was an increase in the percentage of $Foxp3^{+}$ CD25High $CD4^{+}$ cells that expressed CTLA-4 [53].

An additional mechanism is the bystander activation. This is the activation of autoreactive lymphocytes by antigen presenting cells in a proinflammatory environment [54]. This kind of autoreactive T cells activation has been described in Chagas'disease [55].

2.2.3. *Humoral adaptative immunity*

The importance of humoral immunity in controlling *T. cruzi* acute infection has been clearly established. Mice lacking B lymphocytes rapidly succumb to infection [56]. But the fact that attracted most attention from researchers is the production of a wide variety of autoantibodies.

The first autoantibody to be described was one that reacted to endocardium, blood vessels and interstitium of skeletal muscle (EVI) [57], but was the same group of investigators who recognized the heterophil nature of the antibody and realised that had no pathogenic role [58].

Another autoantibody, studied by our group, was anti-laminin antibody [59, 60]. These antibodies were shown to react against *T. cruzi* amastigotes and trypomastigotes and human laminin [61] and deposition of this antibody in marked thickened basement membranes of myocytes, endothelial cells, and vascular smooth muscle cells was shown by us with light microscopy, electron microscopy and immunohistochemical techniques in endomyocardial biopsies of chagasic patients [62] but then we found that only 50% of patients had the antibody on their sera and no correlation with disease severity could be established [59].

Anti-myosin antibodies are postulated by some authors to be generated through molecular mimicry with two *T. cruzi* antigens: B13 protein [63] and cruzipain [64, 65]. Although cruzipain antibodies mainly react to skeletal muscle myosin, they can cause conduction disturbances when transferred to uninfected mice and, when transferred to pregnant animals, they caused conduction disturbances in pups [65]. On the other hand, immunossuppresed mice did not mount any humoral response when immunized with myosin but still develop myocarditis [66].

This fact made some authors doubt on the molecular mimicry hypothesis and rather consider antibodies to myosin a consequence of myocyte damage [67].

Antibodies that react with muscarinic receptors are also being intensely studied. In early 1990's IgG from chagasic patients was observed to bind to muscarinic M2 receptors and activate them [68]. These anti-muscarinic antibodies were found to increase intracellular cGMP and decrease cAMP [69] and were positively related to the presence of dysautonomia [70]. These antibodies also causes accumulation of inositol phosphate and nitric oxide synthase stimulation, with a negative inotropic effect on myocardium [71]. As mentioned before, anti-muscarinic autoantibodies are positively related to the presence of dysautonomia [70], the presence of achalasia in chagasic patients [72], sinus node dysfunction [73], but are not related with the degree of myocardial dysfunction [73, 74], nor with the presence of brain lesions [75]. In fact patients with cardiomyopathy and left ventricular dysfunction but without autonomic dysfunction show low levels of anti-muscarinic antibodies [76].

Autoantibody	Hypothetic pathogenic role	Reference
Anti-Cerebroside	Probably related to neurologial symptoms	[77]
Anti-Gal	Apparently protective	[78]
Anti-Brain Microtubules	Unknown	[79]
Anti-Ribosome	Unknown	[80, 81]
Anti- UsnRNPs	Unkwnown	[82]
Anti-Sulfatides	May cause myocarditis and induce arrhythmias	[83]
Anti-Galectin-1	Increased in CCC patients	[84]
Anti-Cha R3	Specific of CCC	[85]
Anti-Desmoglein-1	Related to Penphigus foliaceum	[86]
Anticardiolipin	Unknown	[87]
Anti- TrkA, TrkB and TrkC	Prevents apoptosis of neurons and helps cellular invasion	[88]
Anti-MBP	Related to gastrointestinal form	[89]

Table 2. Less studied autoantibodies in Chagas' disease

Antibodies against β_1-adrenergic receptors are also intensely studied. Described in early 1980's [90] these antibodies increased cAMP in mouse atrial fibers, increasing the release of PGE_2 and TXB_2 causing diminished contractility [91]. Increased cAMP activates PKA and then increases the intracellular calcium concentration. This causes in turn inhibition of the Na^+/K^+-ATPase and stimulates Ca^{2+}-ATPase activity leading to intracellular depletion of K^+ and further increase in Ca^{2+}. These alteration alter contractility and electric impulse generation and conduction [92]. Antiadrenergic autoantibodies titers could not be related to the severity of left ventricular dysfunction [74] and patients with overt cardiomyopathy but without autonomic dysfunction show low leves of these antibodies [76]. Antibodies against β_2-adrenergic receptors have also been described but are mainly related to megacolon [93].

Antibodies against atrio-ventricular (AV) node and sinus auricular node tissues have been studied as markers of chronic cardiopathy condition. When compared in chronic chagasic cardiopathy patients, non-chagasic cardiopathy patients, indeterminate chagasic subjects, healthy blood donors as controls, they more frequently found in chronic chagasic cardiopathy, but not enough to be good markers for chagasic cardiopathy group. Besides, no clear association with complex rhythm or conduction aberrations was found [94].

Many other autoantibodies have been described (table 2) but are not so widely studied and their role in pathogenesis of chagasic myocarditis is not clear.

2.2.4. Genetic factors

Human Leucocyte Antigen (HLA) have show some relation to de development of CCC. HLA-B40 and Cw3 combination was protective for CCC [95], as resulted DRB1*14, DQB1*0303 [96], HLA-DQB1*06 [97] and HLA-A68 [98]. On the other hand, HLA-C*03 [99], DRB1*1503 [100], DRB1*01, DRB1*08, DQB1*0501 [96] and HLA-DR16 alelles [98] were positively related to the development of CCC.

A number of other genes related to immune system have been studied in order to determine their relation to a predisposition to develop CCC. In table 3 we list those positively related to the appearance of CCC [101].

Gene	Polymorphism
CCL2/MCPI	- 2518
CCR5	+ 53029
TNF-α	- 308G/A, -238G/A, -1031T/C
LT-α	+ 80A/C, + 252A/G
BAT-1	- 22C/G, - 348C/T
NF-kB	- 62, - 262
IL-1β	- 31, + 3954, + 5810
IL-1RN	+11100T/C
IL-4	-509C/T
IL-10	- 1082G/A
IL-12β	+ 1188A/C
INF-γ	+874T/A
MAL/TRIAP	S180L
MCP-1	-2518a/G
MIF	-174G/C
TGF-β1	+10T/C

Table 3. Genetic polymorphisms related to CCC. Adapted from [101, 102].

2.2.5. The cytokines and chemokines

Although proinflammatory cytokines seem to be necessary for controlling parasitemia during acute phase of the disease [101], CCC patients display a rather proinflammatory cytokine while indeterminate patients display a down modulator one. CCC patients have increased levels of

http://dx.doi.org/10.5772/55387

TNF-α and CCL2 than indeterminate patients [103, 104]. Infiltrating macrophages from CCC patients express INF-γ, TNF-α and IL-6 but show low levels of IL-2, IL-4 and IL-10 [105-107]. Also CCR5, CXCR3 and CCR7 and their ligands are increased in hearts of CCC patients, as well as monocytes expressing CXCR3, CCR5, CXCL9 and CCL5 [101]. It has been shown that INF-γ and CCL2 induce myocytes to secrete arial natriuretic factor and cause hyperthrophy [108], and IL-18 and CCR7 ligands, which are increased in CCC, cause cardiomyocyte hyperthrophy and fibrosis [109-111]. Cultures of peripheral blood mononuclear cells from patients with moderate and severe cardiomyopathy produced high levels of TNF-α, IFN-γ and low levels of IL-10, when compared to mild cardiomyopathy or cardiomyopathy-free patients. Flow cytometry analysis showed higher CD4+IL-17+ cells in peripheral blood mononuclear cells cultured from patients without or with mild cardiomyopathy, in comparison to patients with moderate or severe cardiomyopathy, reflecting a relative protective effect of IL-10 and IL-17 compared with INF-γ and TNF-α [112]. In another experiment in which $CD8^+$ in culture were stimulated with trypanosomal antigens, those cells froms patients with CCC produced larger amounts of INF-γ and TNF-α than those obtained from indeterminate patients [113].

2.3. The third ingredient: Fibrosis

Fibrosis is one of the most striking characteristics of CCC. In our experience with endomyocardial biopsies, fibrosis had replaced between 8,2 and 49% of contractile myocardium, with only one patient having less than 10% [49]. In our experience with autopsies of hearts, fibrosis was more extensive in conduction system than in contracting myocardium [2]. The deposition of laminin in extracellular and basement membranes has been implicated in the pathogenesis of inflammatory process, as laminin is able to bind proinflammatory citokines [114]. The inflammatory infiltrate in CCC is related to the production of citokines such as INF-γ, TNF-α, IL-18, CCL2 and CCL21, that may have modulator actions on fibrotic process [101].

3. Pathophysiological consequences of myocarditis

With the perpetuation of inflammation, necrosis and scarring fibrosis, damage to all histological components of myocardium occurs. Damage to contracting myocardial fibers determines contractile failure as well as electrophysiological disturbances. Conduction system, nervous autonomic system and microvasculature are also damaged and as a consequence they cause further damage to contractile myocardium and produce electrical instability.

3.1. Dysautonomia

As early as 1922 Carlos Chagas noted that the chronotropic response to atropine was altered in chagasic patients [115], but it was not until late 1950's that Köberle published his works showing impressive neuronal depopulation in microscopic sections obtained from the intercaval atrial strip in chagasic patients using a standardized technique of cardiac intramural neuronal counting developed by himself [116, 117]. These findings led to the "neurogenic hypothesis" [118], which explained all megas in Chagas' disease as a consequence of neuronal depletion.

Although many other authors claimed to have confirmed this finding [119, 120], other authors called to attention about the criteria used to diagnose neuronal depletion because of the great variability in the number of neurons in autonomic ganglia [121] and they also remark that the only right criterion to establish neuronal depletion is the presence of proliferation of satellite cells, with the formation of Terplan's nodules, a characteristic lesion described as proliferating satellite cells which replace degenerating neurons, forming nodular structures. These lesions, once considered patognomonic, can be found in other cardiomyopathies [121]. The same author could not confirm the loss of neurons or denervation in CCC [122]. Finally, it was demonstrated that, using Terplan's nodules as diagnostic criterion, CCC patients with heart failure has more neuronal depletion than patients with dilated cardiomyopathy of other causes [120]. In our experience the neuroganglionic involvement was variable in autopsies of chagasic hearts [11].

According to neurogenic hypothesis [118], early and irreversible damage to the parasympathetic system during acute phase of the disease causes a cathecolaminergic cardiomyopathy, but this point of view has been debated and evidence is contradictory. Functional test performed in CCC patients demonstrated impaired parasympathetic heart rate regulation: metaraminol, phenylephrine and atropine intravenous injections, facial immersion, Valsalva maneuver, head-up and head-down tilt tests, respiratory sinus arrhythmia, hand grip, graded dynamic exercise, and spectral analysis of Holter recordings [123-130], but a carefull analyasis of these data showed that many patients had normal autonomic function and most patients had heart failure, that could explain autonomic dysfunction per se [131]. But the study of indeterminate patients has shown conflicting results. While some authors could demonstrate impaired autonomic function [132, 133] others could demonstrate that autonomic function was normal in patients without myocardial damage and that abnormalities in autonomic dysfunction was proportional to heart dysfunction, leading these authors to propose that these abnormalities arise as a compensating mechanism for the progressive left ventricular dilatation [134, 135]. These findings led to a new "neurogenic theory", which considers autonomic dysfunction as secondary to ventricular dilatation and hemodynamic alterations, but once installed, acts synergistically with parasitism and inflammation to cause further myocardial damage [136].

3.2. Microvascular damage

Microcirculation abnormalities have been demonstrated in experimental models as well as in clinical practice [137]. Many investigators have found abnormal myocardial perfusion using isonitrile-99m-technetium [138] and thallium-201 [139, 140] scintigraphy in chagasic patients with normal epicardial coronary arteries. Furthermore, the progression of left ventricular systolic dysfunction is associated with both the presence of reversible perfusion defects and the increase in perfusion defects at rest [141, 142]. Anatomopathological studies in humans also provided evidence of microvascular damage in CCC. In late 1950's first reports showing collapse of arterioles and intimal proliferation [143] caught the attention of investigators. Also, microthrombi have been described [144]. In endomyocardial biopsies we also found thickening of capilary basement membranes [49].

Additional evidence of microvascular damage was obtained from experimental models. Vascular constriction, microaneurysm formation, dilatation and proliferation of microvessels has been demonstrated [145-148].

Many factors have been advocated in the genesis of these lesions. First, the parasite itself. It was shown that *T. cruzi* produces a neuraminidase that removes sialic acid from de surface of endotelial cells. This results in thrombin binding and platelet aggregation [149]. *T. cruzi* also produces tromboxane A_2 (TXA_2), specially during amastigote state [150], also favouring platelet aggregation and vascular spasm. Direct parasitism of endothelial cells by *T. cruzi* has also been demonstrated, and this causes the activation of the NF-kB pathway increasing the expression af adhesion molecules [151], and secreting proinflammatory citokines [152] and iNOS [153].

Endothelin-1 (ET-1) is another proposed pathogenic element. Elevated levels of mRNA for preproendothelin-1, endothelin converting enzyme and endothelin-1 were observed in the infected myocardium [154], and elevated levels of ET-1 have been found in CCC patients [155]. Mitogen-activated protein kinases and the transcription factor activator-protein-1 regulate the expression of endothelin-1, and both are shown to be increased in myocardium, interstitial cells and vascular and endocardial endothelial cells [156]. Besides, treatment with phosphoramidon, an inhibitor of endothelin converting enzyme, decreases heart size and severity of pathology in an experimental model of Chagas' disease [157]. Moreover, the use of bosentan, a dual endothelin A (ETA) receptor and endothelin B (ETB) receptor was accompanied by a significant increase in parasitemia and tissue parasitism or inflammation and reduced the infection-associated increase in NOx serum concentration, suggesting that ETA and ETB may play a role in the control of *T. cruzi* infection probably by interfering in NO production [158].

Inflammation also produces dysfunction of endothelial cells. Macrophages secrete TXA_2 and platelet activating factor (PAF) that act on endothelium causing vasoconstriction [159]. Endothelial cells infected *in vitro* with *T. cruzi* lose their antithrombotic properties in response to interleukin 1 β (IL-1β) [160, 161].

It is remarkable that, although the data presented, endothelial function seems to be normal in CCC patients without heart failure, as measured by increases in blood flow in response to acetilcholine and sodium nitroprusside [162]. A normal endothelial function has also been found using pulse plethysmography in 40 asymptomatic patients with Chagas' disease compared with healthy controls, although a prothrombotic and proinflammatory state has been noted in Chagas' disease patients [163].

4. A combined theory that could explain the pathogenic mechanism in chronic chagasic myocarditis

With the perpetuation of inflammation, necrosis and scarring fibrosis, damage to all histological components of myocardium occurs. Damage to contracting myocardial fibers determines contractile failure as well as electrophysiological disturbances. Conduction system, nervous autonomic system and microvasculature are also damaged and as a consequence they cause further damage to contractile myocardium and produce electrical instability. Figure 3 illustrates with a flow chart the interactive network of different elements in the pathogenesis of CCC.

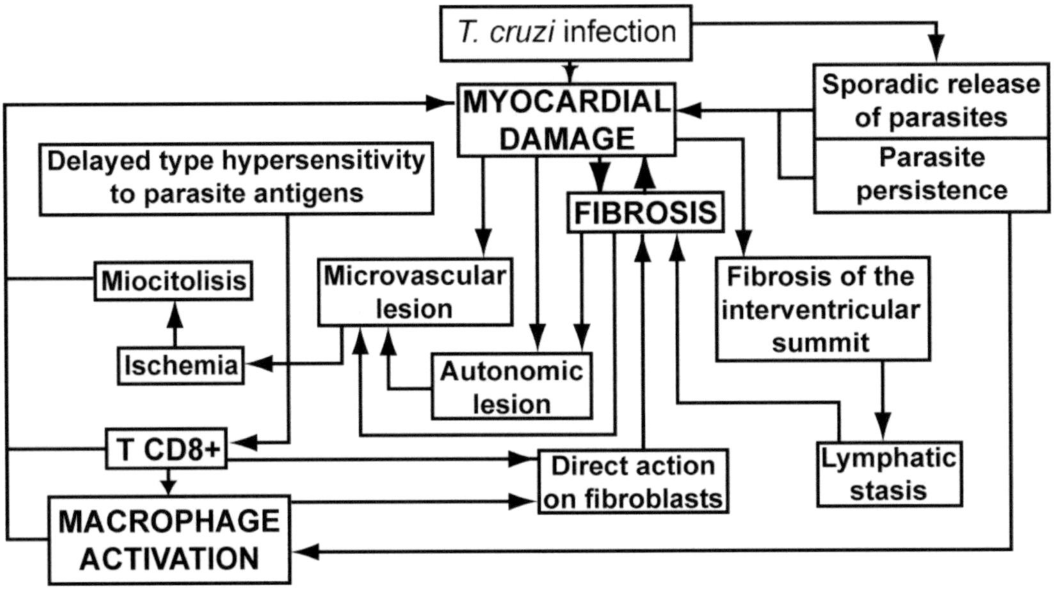

Figure 3. Schematic representation of the integrated theory of multiple factors that determine myocardial damage in CCC.

5. Conclusions

As shown across the sections of this chapter, the numerous hypothesis about pathogenic pathways of CCC have supporting data and pitfalls. All hypothesis finally interact with each other, giving us the idea that none of these theories explains the development of CCC by itself. Rather, it seems more feasible that all of these conform a network of damaging elements, and that all elements cause and/or enhances each other. The triggering element is obviously the interaction between parasite and host's immune system. Cell parasitism, the inflammatory process and consequent necrosis and fibrosis cause damage to contracting myocardium, autonomic system, conduction system and microcirculation. Autonomic damage causes impaired regulation of microvasculature and further alterations in blood flow. Ischemia causes more myocardial damage. Necrosis exposes intracellular epitopes and causes autoantibodies production, with more necrosis, fibrosis and so on. It seems that, if adequate down modulator immune mechanisms work properly, this vicious circle stops and patients do not develop cardiomyopathy, rather they remain in an indeterminate form lifelong.

http://dx.doi.org/10.5772/55387

This work has been performed as part of a Framework Agreement between the Division of Cardiology, University of Perugia, Perugia, Italy, and the Instituto de Investigaciones Cardiológicas "Alberto C. Taquini", University of Buenos Aires, Buenos Aires, Argentina. This study received financial support from PIP 6549, CONICET and UBACYT M052, University of Buenos Aires, Argentina, and from Istituto S. Paolo, Turin, Italy.

Author details

Julián González[1,2], Francisco Azzato[1,2], Giusepe Ambrosio[1,2] and José Milei[1,2]

1 Instituto de Investigaciones Cardiológicas Prof. Dr. A. Taquini – UBA - CONICET, Argentina

2 Division of Cardiology, University of Perugia School of Medicine - Perugia, Italy

References

[1] Guerri-Guttenberg, R.A., et al., *Chagas cardiomyopathy: Europe is not spared!*. European Heart J, 2008. 29(21): p. 2587-2591.

[2] Milei, J., et al., *Myocardial Inflammatory infiltrate in human chronic Chagasic cardiomyopathy: Immunohistochemical findings*. Cardiovasc Pathol, 1996. 5(4): p. 209-219.

[3] Milei, J., et al., *Prognostic impact of Chagas disease in the United States*. American Heart J, 2009. 157(1): p. 22-29.

[4] Milei, J., et al., *Does Chagas' disease exist as an undiagnosd form of cardiomyopathy in the United States?* Am Heart J, 1992. 123(6): p. 1732-1735.

[5] Storino, R.A., H. Barragan, and J. Milei, *Aspectos epidemiologicos de la enfermedad de Chagas en la Argentina y America Latina*. Revista Federación Argentina de Cardiología, 1992. 21(3): p. 239-246.

[6] Chagas, C., *Nova tripanozomiaze humana. Estudos sobre a morfolojia e o ciclo evolutivo do Schizotripannum cruzi n. gen., n. sp., ajente etiolojico de nova entidade mobida do homem*. Memorias do Instituto Oswaldo Cruz, 1909. 1(2): p. 159 - 218.

[7] Rassi, A., Jr., A. Rassi, and J.A. Marin-Neto, *Chagas disease*. Lancet, 2010. 375(9723): p. 1388-402.

[8] WHO, *Reporte sobre enfermedad de Chagas*. 2005.

[9] Rassi, A., Jr., A. Rassi, and W.C. Little, *Chagas' heart disease*. Clinical Cardiology, 2000. 23(12): p. 883-9.

[10] Andrade, Z.A., *A patologia da doenca de Chagas no honen.* Annales de la Societe Belge de Medecine Tropicale, 1985. 65(1): p. 15-30.

[11] Milei, J., et al., *Histopathology of specialized and ordinary myocardium and nerves in chronic Chagas disease, with a morphometric study of inflammation and fibrosis.* Cardiologia, 1991. 36(2): p. 107-115.

[12] Marin-Neto, J.A., et al., *Pathogenesis of Chronic Chagas Heart Disease.* Circulation, 2007. 115(9): p. 1109-1123.

[13] Storino, R.A. and J. Milei, *Enfermedad de Chagas.* 1994, Buenos Aires: Mosby-Doyma. 652.

[14] Gonzalez, J., et al., *Pathogenensis and Pathology of Chronic Chagas' Myocarditis,* in *Myocarditis,* D. Chiakova, Editor. 2011, Intech: Rijeka. p. 119 - 150.

[15] Younées-Chennoufi, A.B., et al., *Persistence of Trypanosoma cruzi antigens in the inflammatory lesions of chronically infected mice.* Trans Roy Soc Trop Med Hyg, 1988. 82: p. 77.

[16] Jones, E.M., et al., *Amplification of Trypanosoma cruzi DNA sequence from inflammatory lesions in human chagasic cardiomyopathy.* Am J Trop Med Hyg, 1993. 48: p. 348-357.

[17] Schijman, A.G., et al., *Trypanosoma cruzi DNA in cardiac lesions of Argentinean patients with end-stage chronic chagas heart disease.* Am J Trop Med Hyg, 2004. 70(2): p. 210-20.

[18] Higuchi, M.L., T. Brito, and M. Martins Reis, *Correlation between trypanosoma cruzi parasitism and myocardial inflammatory infiltrate in human chronic chagasic myocarditis: in light microscopy and immunohistochemical findings.* Cardiovasc Pathol, 1993. 2: p. 101-106.

[19] Añez, N., et al., *Myocardial parasite persistence in chronic chagasic patients.* Amer J Trop Med Hyg, 1999. 60(5): p. 726-732.

[20] Andrade, Z., *Novos aspectos sobre a patogenia da doenca de Chagas.* Rev Soc Bras Med Trop, 1992. 25(3): p. 8.

[21] Basquiera, A.L., et al., *Risk progression to chronic Chagas cardiomyopathy: influence of male sex and of parasitaemia detected by polymerase chain reaction.* Heart, 2003. 89(10): p. 1186-90.

[22] Castro, C., A. Prata, and V. Macedo, *The influence of the parasitemia on the evolution of the chronic Chagas' disease.* Revista da Sociedade Brasileira de Medicina Tropical, 2005. 38(1): p. 1-6.

[23] Tarleton, R. and L. Zhang, *Chagas Disease Etiology: Autoimmunity or Parasite Persistence?* Parasitology Today, 1999. 15(3): p. 94 - 99.

[24] Tyler, K.M. and D.M. Engman, *The life cycle of Trypanosoma cruzi revisited.* International Journal for Parasitology, 2001. 31: p. 472 - 481.

[25] Macedo, A.M., et al., *Trypanosoma cruzi: Genetic Structure of Populations and Relevance of Genetic Variability to the Pathogenesis of Chagas Disease.* Memorias do Instituto Oswaldo Cruz, 2004. 99(1): p. 1 - 12.

[26] Vago, A.R., et al., *Genetic characterization of Trypanosoma cruzi directly from tissues of patients with chronic Chagas disease: differential distribution of genetic types into diverse organs.* The American Journal of Pathology, 2000. 156(5): p. 1805-9.

[27] Yoshida, N. and M.R. Cortez, *Trypanosoma cruzi: parasite and host cell signaling during the invasion process.* Subcellular Biochemistry, ed. R. Harris. Vol. 47. 2008, Houton: Springer Science.

[28] Alves, M.J.M. and W. Colli, *Trypanosoma cruzi: Adhesion to the Host Cell and Intracellular Survival.* IUBMB Life, 2007. 59(4 - 5): p. 274 - 279.

[29] Girones, N., H. Cuervo, and M. Fresno, *Trypanosoma cruzi-induced molecular mimicry and Chagas' disease.* Current Topics in Microbiology and Immunology, 2005. 296: p. 89-123.

[30] Vitelli-Avelar, D.M., et al., *Are increased frequency of macrophage-like and natural killer (NK) cells, together with high levels of NKT and CD4+CD25high T cells balancing activated CD8+ T cells, the key to control Chagas' disease morbidity?* Clinical and Experimental Immunology, 2006. 145(1): p. 81-92.

[31] Brener, Z. and R.T. Gazzinelli, *Immunological control of Trypanosoma cruzi infection and pathogenesis of Chagas' disease.* International Archives of Allergy and Immunology, 1997. 114(2): p. 103-10.

[32] Camargo, M.M., et al., *Glycoconjugates isolated from Trypanosoma cruzi but not from Leishmania species membranes trigger nitric oxide synthesis as well as microbicidal activity in IFN-gamma-primed macrophages.* The Journal of Immunology, 1997. 159(12): p. 6131-6139.

[33] Vitelli-Avelar, D.M., et al., *Chagasic Patients with Indeterminate Clinical Form of the Disease have High Frequencies of Circulating CD3+CD16–CD56+ Natural Killer T Cells and CD4+CD25High Regulatory T Lymphocytes.* Scandinavian Journal of Immunology, 2005. 62(3): p. 297-308.

[34] Sathler-Avelar, R., et al., *Innate immunity and regulatory T-cells in human Chagas disease: what must be understood?* Memorias do Instituto Oswaldo Cruz, 2009. 104 Suppl 1: p. 246-51.

[35] Gomes, J.A., et al., *Evidence that development of severe cardiomyopathy in human Chagas' disease is due to a Th1-specific immune response.* Infection and Immunity, 2003. 71(3): p. 1185-93.

[36] Vitelli-Avelar, D.M., et al., *Strategy to assess the overall cytokine profile of circulating leukocytes and its association with distinct clinical forms of human Chagas disease.* Scandinavian Journal of Immunology, 2008. 68(5): p. 516-25.

[37] de Melo, A.S., et al., *IL-10 and IFN-γ gene expression in chronic Chagas disease patients after in vitro stimulation with recombinant antigens of Trypanosoma cruzi.* Cytokine, 2012. 58(2): p. 207-212.

[38] Gomes, J.A.S., et al., *Impaired phagocytic capacity driven by downregulation of major phagocytosis-related cell surface molecules elicits an overall modulatory cytokine profile in neutrophils and monocytes from the indeterminate clinical form of Chagas disease.* Immunobiology, 2012. 217(10): p. 1005-1016.

[39] Campos, M. and R. Gazzinelli, *Trypanosoma cruzi and its components as exogenous mediators of inflammation recognized through Toll-like receptors.* Mediators of Inflammation, 2004. 13(3): p. 139-143.

[40] Weitzel, T., et al., *Mannose-Binding Lectin and Toll-Like Receptor Polymorphisms and Chagas Disease in Chile.* Am J Trop Med Hyg, 2012. 86(2): p. 229-232.

[41] Cestari, I. and M.I. Ramirez, *Inefficient Complement System Clearance of Trypanosoma cruzi Metacyclic Trypomastigotes Enables Resistant Strains to Invade Eukaryotic Cells.* PloS one, 2010. 5(3): p. e9721.

[42] Boldt, A.B.W., P.R. Luz, and I.J.T. Messias-Reason, *MASP2 haplotypes are associated with high risk of cardiomyopathy in chronic Chagas disease.* Clinical Immunology, 2011. 140(1): p. 63-70.

[43] Dutra, W.O., et al., *Activated T and B lymphocytes in peripheral blood of patients with Chagas' disease.* International Immunology, 1994. 6(4): p. 499-506.

[44] Menezes, C.A.S., et al., *Phenotypic and functional characteristics of CD28+ and CD28− cells from chagasic patients: distinct repertoire and cytokine expression.* Clinical & Experimental Immunology, 2004. 137(1): p. 129-138.

[45] Dutra, et al., *Self and Nonself Stimulatory Molecules Induce Preferential Expansion of CD5+ B Cells or Activated T Cells of Chagasic Patients, Respectively.* Scandinavian Journal of Immunology, 2000. 51(1): p. 91-97.

[46] Souza, P.E.A., et al., *Trypanosoma cruzi Infection Induces Differential Modulation of Costimulatory Molecules and Cytokines by Monocytes and T Cells from Patients with Indeterminate and Cardiac Chagas' Disease.* Infect. Immun., 2007. 75(4): p. 1886-1894.

[47] Souza, P.E., et al., *Monocytes from patients with indeterminate and cardiac forms of Chagas' disease display distinct phenotypic and functional characteristics associated with morbidity.* Infection and Immunity, 2004. 72(9): p. 5283-91.

[48] Villani, F.N., et al., *Trypanosoma cruzi-induced activation of functionally distinct alphabeta and gammadelta CD4- CD8- T cells in individuals with polar forms of Chagas' disease.* Infection and Immunity, 2010. 78(10): p. 4421-30.

[49] Milei, J., et al., *Endomyocardial biopsies in chronic chagasic cardiomyopathy. Immunohistochemical and ultrastructural findings.* Cardiology, 1992. 80(5-6): p. 424-37.

[50] Ribeiro-Dos-Santos, R., et al., *A heart-specific CD4+ T-cell line obtained from a chronic chagasic mouse induces carditis in heart-immunized mice and rejection of normal heart transplants in the absence of Trypanosoma cruzi.* Parasite Immunology, 2001. 23(2): p. 93-101.

[51] Cunha-Neto, E. and J. Kalilf, *Heart-infiltrating and Peripheral T Cells in the Pathogenesis of Human Chagas' Disease Cardiomyopathy.* Autoimmunity, 2001. 34(3): p. 187-192.

[52] Girones, N., et al., *Dominant T- and B-cell epitopes in an autoantigen linked to Chagas' disease.* The Journal of Clinical Investigation, 2001. 107(8): p. 985-93.

[53] de Araújo, F.F., et al., *Regulatory T Cells Phenotype in Different Clinical Forms of Chagas' Disease.* PLoS Neglected Tropical Diseases, 2011. 5(5): p. e992.

[54] Fujinami, R.S., et al., *Molecular Mimicry, Bystander Activation, or Viral Persistence: Infections and Autoimmune Disease.* Clin. Microbiol. Rev., 2006. 19(1): p. 80-94.

[55] Fedoseyeva, E.V., et al., *De Novo Autoimmunity to Cardiac Myosin After Heart Transplantation and Its Contribution to the Rejection Process.* The Journal of Immunology, 1999. 162(11): p. 6836-6842.

[56] Kumar, S. and R.L. Tarleton, *The relative contribution of antibody production and CD8+ T cell function to immune control of Trypanosoma cruzi.* Parasite Immunology, 1998. 20(5): p. 207-216.

[57] Cossio, P.M., et al., *Chagasic Cardiopathy: Demonstration of a Serum Gamma Globulin Factor Which Reacts with Endocardium and Vascular Structures.* Circulation, 1974. 49(1): p. 13-21.

[58] Khoury, E.L., et al., *Heterophil nature of EVI antibody in Trypanosoma cruzi infection.* Clinical Immunology and Immunopathology, 1983. 27(2): p. 283-288.

[59] Milei, J., et al., *Antibodies to laminin and immunohistochemical localization of laminin in chronic chagasic cardiomyopathy: a review.* Molecular and Cellular Biochemistry, 1993. 129(2): p. 161-170.

[60] Sanchez, J.A., et al., *Immunohistochemical localization of laminin in the hearts of patients with chronic chagasic cardiomyopathy: Relationship to thickening of basement membranes.* Am Heart J, 1993. 126: p. 1392-1401.

[61] Szarfman, A., et al., *Antibodies to laminin in Chagas' disease.* The Journal of Experimental Medicine, 1982. 155(4): p. 1161-1171.

[62] Sanchez, J.A., et al., *Immunohistochemical localization of laminin in the hearts of patients with chronic chagasic cardiomyopathy: relationship to thickening of basement membranes.* Am Heart J, 1993. 126(6): p. 1392 - 1401.

[63] Gruber, A. and B. Zingales, *Trypanosoma cruzi: characterization of two recombinant antigens with potential application in the diagnosis of Chagas' disease.* Experimental Parasitology, 1993. 76(1): p. 1-12.

[64] Giordanengo, L., et al., *Cruzipain induces autoimmune response against skeletal muscle and tissue damage in mice.* Muscle & Nerve, 2000. 23(9): p. 1407-1413.

[65] Giordanengo, L., et al., *Induction of antibodies reactive to cardiac myosin and development of heart alterations in cruzipain-immunized mice and their offspring.* European Journal of Immunology, 2000. 30(11): p. 3181-3189.

[66] Neu, N., B. Ploier, and C. Ofner, *Cardiac myosin-induced myocarditis. Heart autoantibodies are not involved in the induction of the disease.* The Journal of Immunology, 1990. 145(12): p. 4094-4100.

[67] Kierszenbaum, F., *Views on the autoimmunity hypothesis for Chagas disease pathogenesis.* FEMS Immunology and Medical Microbiology, 2003. 37(1): p. 1-11.

[68] Sterin-Borda, L., G. Gorelik, and E.S. Borda, *Chagasic IgG binding with cardiac muscarinic cholinergic receptors modifies cholinergic-mediated cellular transmembrane signals.* Clin Immnol Immunopathol, 1991. 61: p. 387-397.

[69] Goin, J., et al., *Interaction of human chagasic IgG with the second extracellular loop of the human heart muscarinic acetylcholine receptor: functional and pathological implications.* The FASEB Journal, 1997. 11(1): p. 77-83.

[70] Goin, J.C., et al., *Identification of antibodies with muscarinic cholinergic activity in human Chagas' disease: pathological implications.* Journal of the Autonomic Nervous System, 1994. 47(1-2): p. 45-52.

[71] Sterin-Borda, L., et al., *Participation of Nitric Oxide Signaling System in the Cardiac Muscarinic Cholinergic Effect of Human Chagasic IgG.* Journal of Molecular and Cellular Cardiology, 1997. 29(7): p. 1851-1865.

[72] Goin, J.C., et al., *Functional implications of circulating muscarinic cholinergic receptor autoantibodies in chagasic patients with achalasia.* Gastroenterology, 1999. 117(4): p. 798-805.

[73] Altschuller, M.B., et al., *Chronic Chagas disease patients with sinus node dysfunction: is the presence of IgG antibodies with muscarinic agonist action independent of left ventricular dysfunction?* Revista da Sociedade Brasileira de Medicina Tropical, 2007. 40(6): p. 665 - 671.

[74] Talvani, A., et al., *Levels of anti-M2 and anti-[beta]1 autoantibodies do not correlate with the degree of heart dysfunction in Chagas' heart disease.* Microbes and Infection, 2006. 8(9-10): p. 2459-2464.

[75] Py, M.O., et al., *The presence of antiautonomic membrane receptor antibodies do not correlate with brain lesions in Chagas' disease.* Arquivos Brasileiros de Cardiologia, 2009. 67(3A): p. 633 - 638.

[76] Sterin-Borda, L. and E. Borda, *Role of Neurotransmitter Autoantibodies in the Pathogenesis of Chagasic Peripheral Dysautonomia.* Annals of the New York Academy of Sciences, 2000. 917(1): p. 273-280.

[77] Avila, J.L. and M. Rojas, *Elevated cerebroside antibody levels in human visceral and cutaneous leishmaniasis, Trypanosoma rangeli infection, and chronic Chagas' disease.* The American Journal of Tropical Medicine and Hygiene, 1990. 43(1): p. 52-60.

[78] Gazzinelli, R.T., *Natural anti-Gal antibodies prevent, rather than cause, autoimmunity in human Chagas' disease.* Research in Immunology, 1991. 142(2): p. 164-7.

[79] Kerner, N., et al., *Trypanosoma cruzi: antibodies to a MAP-like protein in chronic Chagas' disease cross-react with mammalian cytoskeleton.* Experimental Parasitology, 1991. 73(4): p. 451-9.

[80] Levitus, G., et al., *Humoral autoimmune response to ribosomal P proteins in chronic Chagas heart disease.* Clinical and Experimental Immunology, 1991. 85(3): p. 413-7.

[81] Skeiky, Y.A., et al., *Cloning and expression of Trypanosoma cruzi ribosomal protein P0 and epitope analysis of anti-P0 autoantibodies in Chagas' disease patients.* The Journal of Experimental Medicine, 1992. 176(1): p. 201-11.

[82] Bach-Elias, M., et al., *Presence of autoantibodies against small nuclear ribonucleoprotein epitopes in Chagas' patients' sera.* Parasitology Research, 1998. 84(10): p. 796-9.

[83] Garcia, R., et al., *[Anti-sulfatide antibody titers in patients with chronic Chagas disease and other forms of cardiopathy].* Revista Panamericana de Salud Publica, 1998. 3(4): p. 249-56.

[84] Giordanengo, L., et al., *Anti-galectin-1 autoantibodies in human Trypanosoma cruzi infection: differential expression of this beta-galactoside-binding protein in cardiac Chagas' disease.* Clinical and Experimental Immunology, 2001. 124(2): p. 266-73.

[85] Girones, N., et al., *Antibodies to an epitope from the Cha human autoantigen are markers of Chagas' disease.* Clinical and Diagnostic Laboratory Immunology, 2001. 8(6): p. 1039-43.

[86] Diaz, L.A., et al., *Anti-desmoglein-1 antibodies in onchocerciasis, leishmaniasis and Chagas disease suggest a possible etiological link to Fogo selvagem.* The Journal of Investigative Dermatology, 2004. 123(6): p. 1045-51.

[87] Pereira de Godoy, M.R., et al., *Chagas disease and anticardiolipin antibodies in older adults.* Archives of Gerontology and Geriatrics, 2005. 41(3): p. 235-8.

[88] Lu, B., et al., *Autoantibodies to neurotrophic receptors TrkA, TrkB and TrkC in patients with acute Chagas' disease.* Scandinavian Journal of Immunology, 2010. 71(3): p. 220-5.

[89] Oliveira, E.C., et al., *Neuropathy of gastrointestinal Chagas' disease: immune response to myelin antigens.* Neuroimmunomodulation, 2009. 16(1): p. 54-62.

[90] Borda, E., et al., *A circulating IgG in Chagas' disease which binds to beta-adrenoceptors of myocardium and modulates their activity.* Clinical & Experimental Immunology, 1984. 57(3): p. 679 - 686.

[91] Gorelik, G., et al., *Antibodies bind and activate beta adrenergic and cholinergic lymphocyte receptors in Chagas' disease.* Clinical Immunology and Immunopathology, 1990. 55(2): p. 221-36.

[92] Borda, E.S. and L. Sterin-Borda, *Antiadrenergic and mucarinic receptor antibodies in Chagas' cardiomyopathy.* International Journal of Cardiology, 1996. 54: p. 149-156.

[93] Wallukat, G., et al., *Distinct patterns of autoantibodies against G-protein-coupled receptors in Chagas' cardiomyopathy and megacolon. Their potential impact for early risk assessment in asymptomatic Chagas' patients.* Journal of the American College of Cardiology, 2010. 55(5): p. 463-8.

[94] Arce-Fonseca, M., et al., *Autoantibodies to human heart conduction system in Chagas' disease.* Vector Borne and Zoonotic Diseases, 2005. 5(3): p. 233-6.

[95] Llop, E., et al., *[HLA antigens in Chagas cardiomyopathy: new evidence based on a case-control study].* Revista Medica de Chile, 1991. 119(6): p. 633-6.

[96] Fernandez-Mestre, M.T., et al., *Influence of the HLA class II polymorphism in chronic Chagas' disease.* Parasite Immunology, 1998. 20(4): p. 197-203.

[97] Deghaide, N.H., R.O. Dantas, and E.A. Donadi, *HLA class I and II profiles of patients presenting with Chagas' disease.* Digestive Diseases and Sciences, 1998. 43(2): p. 246-52.

[98] Cruz-Robles, D., et al., *MHC class I and class II genes in Mexican patients with Chagas disease.* Human Immunology, 2004. 65(1): p. 60-5.

[99] Layrisse, Z., et al., *HLA-C(*)03 is a risk factor for cardiomyopathy in Chagas disease.* Human Immunology, 2000. 61(9): p. 925-9.

[100] Garcia Borras, S., et al., *Distribution of HLA-DRB1 alleles in Argentinean patients with Chagas' disease cardiomyopathy.* Immunological Investigations, 2009. 38(3-4): p. 268-75.

[101] Cunha-Neto, E., et al., *Immunological and non-immunological effects of cytokines and chemokines in the pathogenesis of chronic Chagas disease cardiomyopathy.* Memorias do Instituto Oswaldo Cruz, 2009. 104 Suppl 1: p. 252-8.

[102] Vasconcelos, R.H.T., et al., *Genetic susceptibility to chronic Chagas disease: An overview of single nucleotide polymorphisms of cytokine genes.* Cytokine, 2012. 59(2): p. 203-208.

[103] Ferreira, R.C., et al., *Increased plasma levels of tumor necrosis factor-alpha in asymptomatic/"indeterminate" and Chagas disease cardiomyopathy patients.* Mem Inst Oswaldo Cruz, 2003. 98(3): p. 407-11.

[104] Talvani, A., et al., *Elevated concentrations of CCL2 and tumor necrosis factor-alpha in chagasic cardiomyopathy.* Clin Infect Dis, 2004. 38(7): p. 943-50.

[105] Reis, D.D., et al., *Characterization of inflammatory infiltrates in chronic chagasic myocardial lesions: presence of tumor necrosis factor-alpha+ cells and dominance of granzyme A+, CD8+ lymphocytes.* Am J Trop Med Hyg, 1993. 48(5): p. 637-44.

[106] Abel, L.C., et al., *Chronic Chagas' disease cardiomyopathy patients display an increased IFN-gamma response to Trypanosoma cruzi infection.* Journal of Autoimmunity, 2001. 17(1): p. 99-107.

[107] Reis, M.M., et al., *An in situ quantitative immunohistochemical study of cytokines and IL-2R+ in chronic human chagasic myocarditis: correlation with the presence of myocardial Trypanosoma cruzi antigens.* Clin Immunol Immunopathol, 1997. 83(2): p. 165-72.

[108] Cunha-Neto, E., et al., *Cardiac gene expression profiling provides evidence for cytokinopathy as a molecular mechanism in Chagas' disease cardiomyopathy.* The American Journal of Pathology, 2005. 167(2): p. 305-13.

[109] Reddy, V.S., et al., *Interleukin-18 stimulates fibronectin expression in primary human cardiac fibroblasts via PI3K-Akt-dependent NF-kappaB activation.* J Cell Physiol, 2008. 215(3): p. 697-707.

[110] Riol-Blanco, L., et al., *The chemokine receptor CCR7 activates in dendritic cells two signaling modules that independently regulate chemotaxis and migratory speed.* J Immunol, 2005. 174(7): p. 4070-80.

[111] Sakai, N., et al., *Secondary lymphoid tissue chemokine (SLC/CCL21)/CCR7 signaling regulates fibrocytes in renal fibrosis.* Proc Natl Acad Sci USA, 2006. 103(38): p. 14098-103.

[112] Guedes, P.M.M., et al., *Deficient Regulatory T Cell Activity and Low Frequency of IL-17-Producing T Cells Correlate with the Extent of Cardiomyopathy in Human Chagas' Disease.* PLoS Neglected Tropical Diseases, 2012. 6(4): p. e1630.

[113] Lorena, V.M.B., et al., *Cytokine Levels in Serious Cardiopathy of Chagas Disease After In Vitro Stimulation with Recombinant Antigens from Trypanosoma cruzi.* Scandinavian Journal of Immunology, 2010. 72(6): p. 529-539.

[114] Savino, W., et al., *Cytokines and cell adhesion receptors in the regulation of Immunity to Trypanosoma cruzi.* Cytokine & Growth Factor Reviews, 2007. 18: p. 107 - 124.

[115] Chagas, C. and E. Vilella, *Cardiac form of American trypanosomiasis.* . Memorias do Instituto Oswaldo Cruz, 1922. 14(1): p. 5 - 61.

[116] Köberle, F., *Chagas disease: a disease of the peripheral autonomic nervous system.* Wien Klin Woschenschr, 1956. 68(17): p. 333 - 339.

[117] Köberle, F., *Pathological findings in muscular hollow organs in experimental Chagas disease.* Zentralbl Allg Pathol, 1956. 95(7 - 8): p. 321 - 329.

[118] Köberle, F., *Cardiopathia parasympathicopriva.* Munch Med Wochenschr, 1959. 101: p. 1308-10.

[119] Mott, K.E. and J.W.C. Hagstrom, *The Pathologic Lesions of the Cardiac Autonomic Nervous System in Chronic Chagas' Myocarditis.* Circulation, 1965. 31(2): p. 273-286.

[120] Oliveira, J.S., *A natural human model of intrinsic heart nervous system denervation: Chagas' cardiopathy.* American Heart Journal, 1985. 110(5): p. 1092 - 1098.

[121] Rossi, L., et al., *Depleción neuronal en la enfermedad de Chagas: todo debería revisarse.* Revista Argentina de Cardiología, 1994. 62(3): p. 239 - 246.

[122] Rossi, L., *Neuroanatomopathology of the cardiovascular system.*, in *Neurocardiology.*, H.E. Kulbertus and G. Franck, Editors. 1988, Futura Publishing Co. Inc.: Mount Kisco, N.Y.

[123] Amorim, D.S., et al., *Effects of acute elevation in blood pressure and of atropine on heart rate in Chagas' disease. A preliminary report.* Circulation, 1968. 38(2): p. 289-94.

[124] Amorim, D.S., et al., *Chagas' heart disease. First demonstrable correlation between neuronal degeneration and autonomic impairment.* Acta Cardiol, 1973. 28(4): p. 431-40.

[125] Manço, J.C., et al., *Degeneration of the cardiac nerves in Chagas' disease. Further studies.* Circulation, 1969. 40(6): p. 879-85.

[126] Marin-Neto, J.A., et al., *Postural reflexes in chronic Chagas's heart disease. Heart rate and arterial pressure responses.* Cardiology, 1975. 60(6): p. 343-57.

[127] Gallo, L., Jr., et al., *Abnormal heart rate responses during exercise in patients with Chagas' disease.* Cardiology, 1975. 60(3): p. 147-62.

[128] Junqueira Junior, L.F., et al., *Subtle cardiac autonomic impairment in Chagas' disease detected by baroreflex sensitivity testing.* Braz J Med Biol Res, 1985. 18(2): p. 171-8.

[129] Guzzetti, S., et al., *Impaired heart rate variability in patients with chronic Chagas' disease.* Am Heart J, 1991. 121(6 Pt 1): p. 1727-34.

[130] Sousa, A.C., et al., *Cardiac parasympathetic impairment in gastrointestinal Chagas' disease.* Lancet, 1987. 1(8539): p. 985.

[131] Davila, D.F., G. Inglessis, and C.A. Mazzei de Davila, *Chagas' heart disease and the autonomic nervous system.* Int J Cardiol, 1998. 66(2): p. 123-7.

[132] Vasconcelos, D.F. and L.F. Junqueira, Jr., *Distinctive impaired cardiac autonomic modulation of heart rate variability in chronic Chagas' indeterminate and heart diseases.* Journal of Electrocardiology, 2009. 42(3): p. 281-9.

[133] Molina, R.B.G., et al., *Dysautonomia and ventricular dysfunction in the indeterminate form of Chagas disease.* International Journal of Cardiology, 2006. 113(2): p. 188-193.

[134] Davila, D.F., et al., *Cardiac parasympathetic innervation in Chagas' heart disease.* Medical Hypotheses, 1991. 35(2): p. 80-4.

[135] Davila Spinetti, D.F., G. Inglessis, and C.A. Mazzei de Davila, *[Chagas cardiomyopathy and the autonomic nervous system. Clinical studies]*. Archivos del Instituto de Cardiologia de Mexico, 1999. 69(1): p. 35-9.

[136] Davila, D.F., et al., *A modified and unifying neurogenic hypothesis can explain the natural history of chronic Chagas heart disease.* International Journal of Cardiology, 2004. 96(2): p. 191-5.

[137] Rossi, M.A., et al., *Coronary Microvascular Disease in Chronic Chagas Cardiomyopathy Including an Overview on History, Pathology, and Other Proposed Pathogenic Mechanisms.* PLoS Neglected Tropical Diseases, 2010. 4(8): p. e674.

[138] Castro, R., E. Kuschnir, and H. Sgammini, *Evaluación de la performance cardíaca y perfusión miocárdica con radiotrazadores en la cardiopatía chagásica crónica.* Revista de la Federación Argentina de Cardiología, 1988. 17: p. 226 - 231.

[139] Marin-Neto, J.A., et al., *Myocardial perfusion abnormalities in chronic Chagas' disease as detected by thallium-201 scintigraphy.* The American Journal of Cardiology, 1992. 69(8): p. 780-4.

[140] Hagar, J.M. and S.H. Rahimtoola, *Chagas' Heart Disease in the United States.* New England Journal of Medicine, 1991. 325(11): p. 763-768.

[141] Hiss, F.C., et al., *Changes in myocardial perfusion correlate with deterioration of left ventricular systolic function in chronic Chagas' cardiomyopathy.* JACC. Cardiovascular Imaging, 2009. 2(2): p. 164-72.

[142] Schwartz, R.G. and O. Wexler, *Early Identification and Monitoring Progression of Chagas' Cardiomyopathy With SPECT Myocardial Perfusion Imaging.* JACC: Cardiovascular Imaging, 2009. 2(2): p. 173-175.

[143] Torres, C.M., *Miocitólise e fibrose do miocárdio na doença de Chagas.* Memorias do Instituto Oswaldo Cruz, 1960. 58(2): p. 161 - 182.

[144] Rossi, M.A., S. Gonçalves, and R. Ribeiro-dos-Santos, *Experimental Trypanosoma cruzi Cardiomyopathy in BA4LB/c Mice. The Potential Role of Intravascular Platelet Aggregation in its Genesis.* American Journal of Pathology, 1984. 114(2): p. 209 - 216.

[145] Factor, S.M. and E.H. Sonnenblick, *Hypothesis: Is congestive cardiomyopathy caused by a hyperreactive myocardial microcirculation (Microvascular spasm)?* The American Journal of Cardiology, 1982. 50(5): p. 1149-1152.

[146] Morris, S.A., et al., *Verapamil ameliorates clinical, pathologic and biochemical manifestations of experimental chagasic cardiomyopathy in mice.* Journal of the American College of Cardiology, 1989. 14(3): p. 782-789.

[147] Tanowitz, H.B., et al., *Parasitic diseases of the heart I: Acute and chronic Chagas' disease.* Cardiovascular Pathology, 1992. 1(1): p. 7-15.

[148] Tanowitz, H.B., et al., *Compromised Microcirculation in Acute Murine Trypanosoma cruzi Infection.* The Journal of Parasitology, 1996. 82(1): p. 124 - 130.

[149] Libby, P., J. Alroy, and M.E. Pereira, *A neuraminidase from Trypanosoma cruzi removes sialic acid from the surface of mammalian myocardial and endothelial cells.* The Journal of Clinical Investigation, 1986. 77(1): p. 127-135.

[150] Ashton, A.W., et al., *Thromboxane A2 is a key regulator of pathogenesis during Trypanosoma cruzi infection.* The Journal of Experimental Medicine, 2007. 204(4): p. 929-940.

[151] Huang, H., et al., *Infection of Endothelial Cells with Trypanosoma cruzi Activates NF-kappa B and Induces Vascular Adhesion Molecule Expression.* Infect. Immun., 1999. 67(10): p. 5434-5440.

[152] Tanowitz, H.B., et al., *Cytokine Gene Expression of Endothelial Cells Infected with Trypanosoma cruzi.* Journal of Infectious Diseases, 1992. 166(3): p. 598-603.

[153] Huang, H., et al., *Expression of Cardiac Cytokines and Inducible Form of Nitric Oxide Synthase (NOS2) inTrypanosoma cruzi-infected Mice.* Journal of Molecular and Cellular Cardiology, 1999. 31(1): p. 75-88.

[154] Petkova, S.B., et al., *Myocardial Expression of Endothelin-1 in Murine Trypanosoma cruzi Infection.* Cardiovascular Pathology, 2000. 9(5): p. 257-265.

[155] Salomone, O.A., et al., *High plasma immunoreactive endothelin levels in patients with Chagas' cardiomyopathy.* The American Journal of Cardiology, 2001. 87(10): p. 1217-1220.

[156] Petkova, S.B., et al., *The role of endothelin in the pathogenesis of Chagas' disease.* International Journal for Parasitology, 2001. 31(5-6): p. 499-511.

[157] Jelicks, L.A., et al., *Cardioprotective effects of phosphoramidon on myocardial structure and function in murine Chagas' disease.* International Journal for Parasitology, 2002. 32(12): p. 1497-506.

[158] Rachid, M.A., et al., *Blockade of endothelin ETA/ETB receptors favors a role for endothelin during acute Trypanosoma cruzi infection in rats.* Microbes and Infection, 2006. 8(8): p. 2113-2119.

[159] Rossi, M.A. and S.G. Carobrez, *Experimental Trypanosoma cruzi cardiomyopathy in BALB/c mice: histochemical evidence of hypoxic changes in the myocardium.* British Journal of Experimental Pathology, 1985. 66(2): p. 155 - 160.

[160] Bevilacqua, M.P., et al., *Interleukin 1 (IL-1) induces biosynthesis and cell surface expression of procoagulant activity in human vascular endothelial cells.* The Journal of Experimental Medicine, 1984. 160(2): p. 618-623.

[161] Nachman, R.L., et al., *Interleukin 1 induces endothelial cell synthesis of plasminogen activator inhibitor.* The Journal of Experimental Medicine, 1986. 163(6): p. 1595-1600.

[162] Consolim-Colombo, F.M., et al., *Endothelial Function Is Preserved in Chagas' Heart Disease Patients Without Heart Failure.* Endothelium, 2004. 11(5-6): p. 241-246.

[163] Herrera, R.N., et al., *Inflammatory and Prothrombotic Activation With Conserved Endothelial Function in Patients With Chronic, Asymptomatic Chagas Disease.* Clinical and Applied Thrombosis/Hemostasis, 2011. 17(5): p. 502-507.

Chapter 6

Peripartum Myocarditis

Marina Deljanin Ilic and Dejan Simonovic

Additional information is available at the end of the chapter

http://dx.doi.org/10.5772/54778

1. Introduction

Cardiac disease in pregnancy is a leading cause of maternal and neonatal morbidity and mortality [1]. Pregnancy not only poses a risk of maternal mortality but also of serious morbidity such as heart failure, stroke and cardiac arrhythmias. Heart failure during pregnancy was recognized as early as 19th century [2], however, the syndrome was not recognized as a distinct clinical entity until the 1937, when Gouley et al. [3] described the clinical and pathologic features of seven pregnant women who had severe and often fatal heart failure. In 1971, Demakis et al. [4] described 27 patients who presented during the puerperium with cardiomegaly, abnormal electrocardiographic findings, and congestive heart failure, and named the syndrome peripartum cardiomyopathy (PPCM). The European Society of Cardiology [5] recently defined peripartum cardiomyopathy as an idiopathic cardiomyopathy presenting with heart failure secondary to left ventricular systolic dysfunction towards the end of pregnancy or in the months following delivery, where no other cause of heart failure is found. It is a diagnosis of exclusion. The left ventricle may not be dilated but the ejection fraction is nearly always reduced below 45%.

The etiology of this disease remains uncertain, but a number of possible causes of PPCM have been proposed [5], including myocarditis, abnormal immune response to pregnancy, maladaptive response to the hemodynamic stress of pregnancy, stress activated cytokines, viral infection, and prolonged tocolysis. In addition, there have been a few reports of familial PPCM [6 - 8], raising the possibility that some cases of PPCM are actually familial dilated cardiomyopathy unmasked by pregnancy. Overall, there is more evidence to support myocarditis or an autoimmune process as the cause of the disease than for other proposed etiologies.

The beginning of the myocarditis hypothesis is related to work of Gouley et al. [3], who reported several cases of heart failure in women dying in the puerperium. Also, they found enlarged hearts with focal areas of necrosis and fibrosis and they also proposed infection as a possible cause of heart failure in these women. After that, Melvin and colleagues proposed myocarditis as the cause for PPCM and reported a dense lymphocyte infiltrate with variable amounts of myocyte oedema, necrosis, and fibrosis in right ventricular biopsy specimens. They also noted that treatment with prednisone and azathioprine resulted in clinical improvement and loss of inflammatory infiltrate on repeated biopsies in the three patients studied [9,10]. Rizeq et al. [11] also found an inflammatory component in less than 10% of biopsy samples from patients with PPCM, a proportion similar to that found in age-and-sex-matched patients with idiopathic dilated cardiomyopathy. The highest frequency of myocarditis (78%) was reported by Midei et al., who found 14 of the 18 patients to have borderline and/or established histologic myocarditis. In that study resolution of myocarditis was associated with improved left ventricular function in the post-partum period [12]. A decade later, Felker and colleagues [13] confirmed that the absence or presence of inflammation on endomyocardial biopsy tissue did not predict outcome in patients with PPCM. However in that endomyocardial biopsy study, the authors also showed a high incidence of active viral myocarditis, using the Dallas criteria, in 26 of 51 PPCM patients. Bultmann et al. [14] found that after a viral infection, a pathologic immune response might occur that is inappropriately directed against native cardiac tissue proteins, leading to ventricular dysfunction. However, in that study the same incidence and types of viral positivity were noted also in controls.

Why should myocarditis be more common in pregnancy? It is assumed that the amended or muted immune response during pregnancy allows viral replication and greater likelihood of myocarditis in the setting of a viral infection [15]. Also it is known that pregnancy results in an immuno compromised state and that the decreased humoral and cellular immunity in pregnancy, together with higher levels of corticosteroids, and raised titres of 'blocking antibodies' formed in normal pregnancy, may allow greater viral replication than in age-matched non-pregnant individuals, and thus, a greater probability of viral myocarditis in the context of infection [16,17].

Farber and Glasgow [16] in their animal studies demonstrated that pregnant mice are more susceptible to viral infections than non-pregnant ones. Furthermore, they found that these viruses multiply to a greater level in the hearts of pregnant mice. The physiologic and hemodynamic changes of pregnancy may result in an increased susceptibility to viral myocarditis, higher virus load (such as coxsackie and echoviruses), and worsening of myocardial viral lesions [16, 17]. Pregnancy may predispose women to a more severe form of viral myocarditis when they are infected by a cardiotropic virus [18]. Immunologic studies in women have demonstrated enhanced suppressor cell activity during pregnancy [19], which could augment susceptibility to viral infections [20, 21].

2. Pathogenesis

2.1. Infection

Myocarditis is the term used to indicate acute infective, toxic or autoimmune inflammation of the heart [22]. It can be caused by many different viruses and the microbial pathogenesis may

http://dx.doi.org/10.5772/54778

be complex. Myocardial inflammatory reaction can be directed against the specific virus infection or predominantly reflects local autoimmune processes. Probably combination of autoimmune processes and virus-associated pathogenicity determines the outcome of the disease. A wide spectrum of agents has been associated with myocarditis, and the more common of these are listed in Table 1.

Etiology	Examples
Infectious	Adenovirus, Coxsackievirus, Cytomegalovirus, Epstein–Barr virus, HIV-1, Borrelia (Lyme's disease), Toxoplasmosis, Actimonices, Chlamydia, Coxiella burneti, Echinococcus granulosus
Drug induced	Amphetamines, Anthracyclines (especially doxorubicin), Catecholamines, Cocaine, Cyclophosphamid, Trastuzumab
Systemic diseases (autoimmune disease)	Crohn's disease, Kawasaki disease, Sarcoidosis, Ulcerative colitis, Cardiac rejection, Peri-partum myocarditis, Giant cell myocarditis, Systemic lupus erythematosus, Dermatomyositis
Hypersensitivity to drugs	Hydrochlorothiazide and loop diuretics, Methyldopa Penicillin, Ampicilin, Sulphadiazine, Sulphamethoxazole

HIV - human immunodeficiency virus

Table 1. Common etiology of myocarditis

During the acute viremic stage, viral replication can be present, in the absence of significant host immune responses. Viruses can enter the cardiac myocytes, fibroblasts, or endothelial cells through receptor-mediated endocytosis. Acute myocardial injury can result from either direct virus-mediated lytic processes or is caused by the emerging antiviral immune response. In fulminant cases of myocarditis, resulting myocyte necrosis may cause a significant loss of contractile tissue, which is accompanied by rapidly developing heart failure and early death of the host. It seems that the virus enters cardiomyocytes or macrophages via specific receptors and coreceptors. For example, a receptor for the coxsackie and adenoviruses 2 and 5 is the coxsackie adenoviral receptor [23]. Coreceptor has a role in serotypes B1, B2, and B5, and it is estimated that this activation may play a role of coreceptor acceleration and can cause an increase in virulence of Coxsackie virus B3. Virulence of Coxsackie virus B3 depends on the viral genome, as well as a host of factors, which may be increased by deficient levels of selenium or copper [24]. During the second stage of infection initial immune response is essential in defending the body during early infection. Natural killer cells and macrophages cause cytokine production (tumor necrosis factor-α, interleukin-1, interleukin-2, and interferon gamma) and inflammatory cell infiltration of the myocardium. The third stage consists of fibrotic reparation and cardiac dilatation in the presence or absence of low-level persistent viral genomes [25]. Important place of myocarditis pathogenesis belongs to the mechanism of molecular mimicry, which means that the activated T killer cells are not just attacking viruses and viral antigens, but they can function on their own proteins, in this case myosin. Further activation of B cells leads to production of specific antibodies as a central place in the subacute and chronic phase of myocarditis. This leads to further necrosis, fibrosis, cardiac remodeling, dilatation, and chronic heart failure (figure 1).

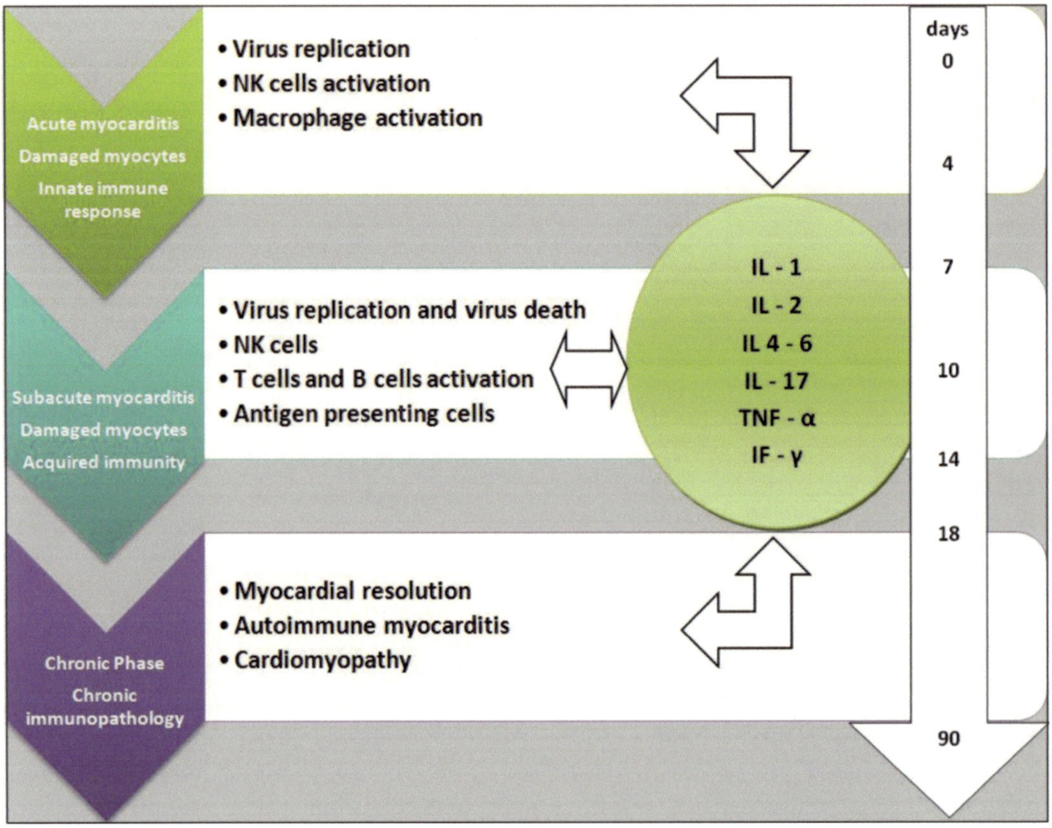

Figure 1. Transition from inflammation to cardiomyopathy

Because of the myocarditis-like inflammatory response seen in endomyocardial biopsy specimens (EMBs) from patients with PPCM, a possibility is reactivation of latent virus infection as a consequence of impaired immune mechanisms during pregnancy [26]. However, no investigation regarding the prevalence of viral genomes in PPCM has been published until recently, when endomyocardial biopsy specimens from 26 patients with PPCM revealed viral genomes (parvovirus B19, human herpes virus 6, Epstein–Barr virus, and human cytomegalovirus) in 8 patients (30.7%) that were associated immunohistologically with interstitial inflammation [14]. The presence of viral genomes in EMBs was associated with inflammatory cardiomyopathy exclusively in patients with PPCM but not in control subjects. Bachmaier et al. [27] reported experimental data supporting the Chlamydia hypothesis. A peptide from the murine heart muscle-specific alpha myosin heavy chain that has sequence homology to the 60-kDa cysteine-rich outer membrane proteins of Chlamydia pneumoniae, Chlamydia psittaci and Chlamydia trachomatis was shown to induce autoimmune inflammatory heart disease in mice. Injection of the homologous Chlamydia peptides into mice also induced perivascular inflammation, fibrotic changes and blood vessel occlusion in the heart. Chlamydia DNA functioned as an adjuvant in the triggering of peptide-induced inflammatory heart disease. In the study of Cenac et al. [28], 96% of patients with PPCM versus 80% of controls were positive for Chlamydia IgG antibodies.

3. Autoimmune mechanisms

The introduction of fetal cells of hematopoietic origin into the maternal circulation may have a significant influence on the immune and genetic alterations. In women with PPCM, high titers of autoantibodies against select cardiac tissue proteins (adenine nucleotide translocator, branched chain α-keto acid dehydrogenase) and increased levels of tumor necrosis factor-alpha, interleukin- 6, and soluble Fas receptors (an apoptosis signaling receptor) have been reported, suggesting a possible role of abnormal immunologic activities and inflammatory cytokines in pathogenesis of this disease [29-31].

The serum from women with peripartum cardiomyopathy has been found to contain autoantibodies in high titers, which are not present in serum from patients with idiopathic cardiomyopathy [32]. Most of these antibodies are against normal human cardiac tissue proteins of 37, 33, and 25 kD. The peripheral blood in these patients has a high level of fetal microchimerism in mononuclear cells, an abnormal cytokine profile, and low levels of CD4+ CD25lo regulatory T cells. Some authors postulated that after delivery the fast degeneration of the uterus results in fragmentation of tropocollagen by collagenolytic enzymes releasing actin, myosin, and their metabolites [33]. Antibodies are formed against actin that cross-react with the myocardium, and the patient subsequently has a cardiomyopathy.

4. Prevalence and clinical features

The prevalence of acute peripartum myocarditis is unknown because most cases are not recognized on account of non-specific, only mild, or no symptoms, but sudden death may occur [22]. The clinical manifestations of myocarditis are various. Myocarditis may develop as a complication of an upper respiratory or gastrointestinal infection with general symptoms, particularly fever and skeletal myalgia, malaise, and anorexia. Since myocarditis may not develop for several days or weeks after symptoms and after return to a normal activity, there is a risk of overexertion, which may be dangerous. Arrhythmias or conduction disturbances may be life threatening despite only mild focal injury, whereas more widespread inflammation is necessary before cardiac dysfunction can cause symptoms.

The initial presentation may be with heart failure or suspected acute myocardial infarction. Acute onset of chest pain is usual and may mimic myocardial infarction or be associated with pericarditis. Symptoms resembling those of heart failure such as dyspnea, dizziness, ankle edema, and orthopnea can occur even in normal pregnancies. Therefore, a pregnant woman in whom peripartum myocarditis and/or cardiomyopathy is developing may consider her symptoms to be normal. If swelling and other heart failure symptoms develop suddenly in an otherwise normal pregnancy, this should prompt further investigation.

5. Investigations

The initial evaluation of acute peripartum myocarditis includes detailed history and careful physical examination.

The ECG is not specific for diagnosis, but it may show sinus tachycardia, focal or generalised abnormalities, ST-segment elevation, fascicular blocks or atrioventricular conduction disturbances [34]. Although the ECG abnormalities are non-specific, an abnormal ECG maydraw attention to the heart and lead to other investigations.

The chest *x* ray may be normal, or show cardiac enlargement, pulmonary venous congestion or pleural effusions.

There is no specific serum marker for myocarditis. Laboratory tests may show leukocytosis, elevated erythrocyte sedimentation rate, eosinophilia, or an elevation in the cardiac fraction of creatine kinase. Evidence of myocyte necrosis may be found with an increase in creatine kinase or appearance of troponin, indicating myocytolysis. The highest enzyme concentrations occur early and will probably have returned to normal by about a week after onset [35].

Cardiac autoantibodies can be demonstrated only late in the disease process, and a viral origin of myocarditis can only be proved if the virus is detected within an altered myocardium. Levels of BNP do not change significantly during normal pregnancy or in the postpartum period, but are markedly elevated in patients with peripartum cardiomyopathy [36]. So, an early measurement of BNP could help in detection of systolic dysfunction and elevation of left ventricle end-diastolic pressure.

Echocardiography may reveal segmental or generalised wall motion abnormalities, left ventricular dilatation, or a pericardial effusion. Echocardiography allows other causes of heart failure to be excluded but pronounced focal changes in wall motion may lead to confusion with myocardial infarction, especially if the ECG changes also suggest this [37]. The advent of novel echocardiographic techniques provides the opportunity to study peripartum myocarditis further. These techniques include those for studying ventricular long-axis function, right ventricular function, tissue Doppler techniques including strain and strain rate echocardiography, and speckle tracking echocardiography. New echo technologies, mainly three-dimensional echocardiography (3DE) and speckle tracking echocardiography, have become available and are competitive with cardiac magnetic resonance imaging (MRI) in accuracy while being less expensive and more widely available [38]. Unfortunately, these novel techniques have not been widely utilized to study peripartum myocarditis and PPCM.

Cardiac magnetic resonance imaging has been recently developed for the diagnosis of myocarditis. It allows more accurate measurement of chamber volumes and global and segmental myocardial function than echocardiography has a higher sensitivity for the detection of LV thrombus [39], and it can characterize the myocardium [40]. In suspected myocarditis MRI can localize and quantify tissue injury, including edema, hyperemia, and fibrosis. In recent series of 82 patients with myocarditis who had biopsy-proven disease, MRI alone made the correct diagnosis in 80% cases [41].There are limited data during organogenesis available, but MRI is probably safe, especially after the first trimester [42].

In the acute phase, the use of contrast media such as gadolinium-diethylene triamino pentaacetic acid (gadolinium-DTPA) helps to differentiate accurately healthy from inflamed or injured tissue. Furthermore, delayed contrast enhancement with gadolinium can help differentiate the type of myocyte necrosis: myocarditis vs ischemia. Myocarditis has a nonvascular distribution in the subepicardium with a nodular or band-like pattern, whereas ischemia has a vascular distribution in a subendocardial or transmural location [43]. Gadolinium can be assumed to cross the fetal blood–placental barrier, but data are limited. The long-term risks of exposure of the developing fetus to free gadolinium ions are not known, and therefore gadolinium during pregnancy should be avoided, but after delivery it represents a useful method for myocarditis diagnosis. Breast feeding does not need to be interrupted after administration of gadolinium [44,45] The importance of MRI is the fact that it is a non-invasive method, there is no risk unlike endomyocardial biopsy, and it can be used to monitor the effects of therapy.

The diagnostic gold standard is endomyocardial biopsy (EMB) with the histological Dallas criteria [46, 47] in conjunction with the new tools of immunohistochemistry and viral polymerase chain reaction (PCR). EMB and PCR are particularly important for those patients who are not experiencing improvement in the early weeks after the diagnosis and therapy, since emerging new antiviral and immunomodulatory treatments depend upon knowing if virus is present or absent in cardiac tissue. It is recommended that MRI should be performed before taking tissue samples, to reduce the sampling error. Leurent et al. [48] advocate using cardiac MRI to guide biopsy to the abnormal area, which may be much more useful than blind biopsy. Whether endomyocardial biopsy should be done in the setting of peripartum myocarditis is still controversial. Some authors not recommend it [49, 50] while Midei et al. [12] recommend endomyocardial biopsy of all patients with peripartum cardiomyopathy and myocarditis who fail to normalize left ventricular function after one week of standard medical therapy.

6. Management

The most important thing in treatment planning is clinical status of the mother and the fetus. If the patient is haemodynamically stable vaginal delivery should be carried out. Urgent delivery irrespective of gestation duration should be considered in women with advanced heart failure and haemodynamic instability despite treatment. Caesarean section is recommended with combined spinal and epidural anaesthesia. An experienced interdisciplinary team is required (cardiologist, obstetrician, anaesthesiologist, neonatologist and intensive care physician) [51].

Heart failure should be treated according to guidelines on heart failure [52], and it can be divided into supportive (heart failure therapy, heart rhythm disturbances, cardiogenic shock), and specific therapy (immunosuppressive therapy, interferon, immunoglobulin, immune-adsorptive therapy, immune-modulation). Heart failure therapy involves administration of diuretics, vasodilators, inotropes, beta blockers, angiotensin-converting enzyme inhibitors (ACEI), angiotensin II receptor blockers (ARBs), anticoagulation therapy, and mechanical support with intraaortic balloon pump or ventricular assist devices in cardiogenic shock as a bridge to recovery or heart transplantation. During pregnancy, ACEI, ARBs and renin inhibitors are contraindicated because they can cause birth defects, although they are the main treatment for postpartum women with heart failure [53, 54]. Digoxin, beta-blockers, loop diuretics, and drugs that reduce afterload such as hydralazine and nitrates have been proven to be safe and are the mainstays of medical therapy of heart failure during pregnancy [15, 55]. Warfarin can cause spontaneous fetal cerebral hemorrhage in the second and third trimesters and therefore is generally contraindicated during pregnancy [56].

7. Specific therapy

In case of early stages of myocarditis, administration of antiviral medications that target viral attachment to host-cell receptors, virus entry, or virus uncoating, would be effective.

Interferon beta. It was shown that beta interferon can decrease the number of viruses up to complete regression, the accumulation of viral RNA and viral coat protein. Interferon beta (IFN-β1a) may affect the elimination of viruses, repair left ventricular ejection fraction and clinical status of patients [57]. In the study of Schmidt-Luce et al. [58], parvovirus B19 and human herpes virus-6 responded less well upon IFN-β treatment with respect to virus clearance and hemodynamic changes, although affected patients can improve clinically, despite incomplete virus clearance following reduction of virus load and/or improvement of endothelial dysfunction. Complete clearance of those viruses may need longer treatment, higher doses, or even change of the antiviral treatment regimens. Currently, there is no approved treatment for chronic viral heart disease, but data have demonstrated that subgroups of patients who had not improved upon regular heart failure medication may get significant benefit even years after onset of chronic disease.

Immunosuppressive therapy. It could be considered in patients with proven myocarditis. Administration of immunosuppressive (corticosteroids, azathioprine, cyclosporine) is still controversial and investigators have emphasized the need to rule out viral infection before starting immunosuppressive treatment, as the treatment may activate a latent virus, with subsequent deterioration in myocardial function [59]. In published randomized study on the Tailored Immunosuppression in Inflammatory Cardiomyopathy (TIMIC study) authors confirmed a positive treatment response in patients with chronic active myocarditis [60]. According to studies performed until now, immunosuppressive therapy should not be routinely administered to patients with myocarditis. However, patients with giant cell myocarditis, autoimmune or hypersensitive myocarditis with heart failure can benefit from this therapy. The best responders may be those with active autoimmune response without persisting viral genome [61].

Immunoglobulin. In case of autoimmune myocarditis, inflammatory process in the myocardium is triggered by a transient viral infection. Instead of anticytokine or immune-suppression therapy, a possible strategy is passive immunization through the infusion of immune globulins. Bozkurt and colleagues added intravenous immune globulin to conventional heart failure therapy in 6 women with PPCM and reported a significantly greater improvement in left ventricular ejection fraction compared with 11 control patients who received conventional therapy alone. Although the results seemed encouraging, a very small number of patients and the lack of a blindly randomized, well-matched control group limited the study [62]. However, McNamara et al. [63] reported that improvement of left ventricular ejection fraction was identical in both the intravenous immuneoglobulin treatment arm and in the placebo arm. These results suggest that for patients with recent-onset dilated cardiomyopathy, immunoglobulins do not improve left ventricular ejection fraction. There are no reliable data for the application of this type of therapy in the adult population with viral myocarditis who do not respond to immunosuppressive therapy [61].

Adsorptive immune therapy. Involves the use of plasmapheresis to remove circulating cytokines and antibodies to cardiomyocytes, beta-adrenergic receptors, adenosintriphosphate carriers, myosin. If this treatment is applied five or more days, beside elimination of circulating antibodies and immune complexes, it also effects the elimination from the heart muscle. Removal of circulating antibodies by immunoadsorption improved cardiac function and clinical and humoral markers of heart failure severity (NT-proBNP) [64]. Immunoadsorption can also decrease myocardial inflammation, and in patients with inflammatory cardiomyopathy, left ventricular systolic function improved after protein A immunoadsorption [65]. The value of adsorptive immune therapy should be confirmed in larger studies.

Monoclonal antibodies. There are some data about possible use of monoclonal antibodies in myocarditis due to T-cell mediated inflammation. Wang et al. [66]. showed that administration of anti-CD4 monoclonal antibody can induce immune tolerance to porcine cardiac myosin. Cardiac function of antibody-treated rats was significantly increased compared with untreated rats 18 days postimmunization examined by transthoracic echocardiography. Also, antibody-treated rats had no proliferative response to porcine cardiac myosin examined by lymphocyte proliferation assay, and administration of anti-CD4 monoclonal antibody significantly prevented production of anti-cardiac myosin antibodies. The conclusion of that study was that immune tolerance to cardiac myosin could be induced by anti-CD4 monoclonal antibody in vivo, and cardiac dysfunction and myocardial injury could be prevented by induction of immune tolerance.

8. Prognosis

Recovery from acute myocarditis often surprises and delights after life threatening illness. Clinical recovery may be slow and delayed even up to a year or more after delivery. Even when it appears to be complete, a portion of cardiovascular reserve has been lost, as is indicated by the myocytolysis found on biopsy [22]. It is also uncertain how many patients will progress to cardiomyopathy. Recurrence in future pregnancies is not invariable, but there are few data. Pregnancy should therefore be discouraged in any woman with residual myocardial dysfunction or, if possible, delayed for some years.

9. Summary

Myocarditis is an inflammatory disease of the myocardium that is diagnosed by histological, immunological and immunochemical criteria, and is associated with cardiac dysfunction. There has been greater evidence for myocarditis as a cause of PPCM than any other proposed aetiological factor. The prevalence of acute peripartum myocarditis is unknown because most cases are not recognized on account of non-specific, only mild, or no symptoms, but sudden death may occur. However, the initial presentation may be with acute or chronic heart failure or mimics acute myocardial infarction. The combination of biomarkers from blood samples together with imaging techniques such as echocardiography and MRI may help to confirm the diagnosis of myocarditis.The diagnostic gold standard is endomyocardial biopsy with the histological Dallas criteria in conjunction with the new tools of immunohistochemistry and viral polymerase chain reaction. Whether endomyocardial biopsy should be done in the setting of peripartum myocarditis is still an open question. The most important thing in treatment planning is clinical status of the mother and the fetus. Heart failure in postpartum women should be treated according to guidelines on heart failure. Pregnant women should not receive angiotensin-converting enzyme inhibitors, angiotensin receptor blockers, or warfarin because of potential teratogenic effects. Specific therapy strategies may include: immunosuppressive therapy, interferon, immunoglobulin, immune-adsorptive therapy, immune-modulation. Subsequent pregnancies carry a high risk of relapse, even in women who have fully recovered left ventricular function.

Author details

Marina Deljanin Ilic[1*] and Dejan Simonovic[2]

*Address all correspondence to: marinadi@open.telekom.rs

1 Institute of Cardiology, Niška Banja, University of Niš Faculty of Medicine, Serbia

2 Institute of Cardiology, Niška Banja, Serbia

References

[1] Gelson E, Johnson M, Gatzoulis M, Uebing A. Review Cardiac disease in pregnancy. Part 2: acquired heart disease. The Obstetrician & Gynaecologist. 2007;9:83–87.

[2] Richie C. Clinical contributions to the pathology, diagnosis, and treatment of certain chronic diseases of the heart. Edinb Med Surg J. 1849; 2: 333.

[3] Gouley BA, McMillan TM, Bellet S. Idiopathic myocardial degeneration associated with pregnancy and especially the puerperium. Am J Med Sci 1937;19:185–99.

[4] Demakis JG, Rahimtoola SH, Sutton GC, et al. Natural course of peripartum cardiomyopathy. Circulation 1971; 44:1053–61.

[5] Sliwa K, Hilfiker-Kleiner D, Petrie MC, et al. Current state of knowledge on aetiology, diagnosis, management, and therapy of peripartum cardiomyopathy: a position statement from the Heart Failure Association of the European Society of Cardiology Working Group on peripartum cardiomyopathy. Eur Heart J 2010; 12: 767–78.

[6] Pierce JA, Price BO, Joyce JW. Familial occurrence of postpartal heart failure. Arch Intern Med 1963;111:651–55.

[7] Pearl W. Familial occurrence of peripartum cardiomyopathy. Am Heart J 1995;129:421–2.

[8] Massad LS, Reiss CK, Mutch DG, Hasket EJ. Family peripartum cardiomyopathy after molar pregnancy. Obstet Gynecol 1993;81:886–88.

[9] Melvin KR, Richardson PJ, Olsen EG, Daly K, Jackson G. Peripartum cardiomyopathy due to myocarditis. N Engl J Med 1982; 307:731–34.

[10] Sanderson JE, Olsen EG, Gatei D. Peripartum heart disease: an endomyocardial biopsy study. Br Heart J 1986; 56:285–91.

[11] Rizeq MN, Rickenbacher PR, Fowler MB, Billingham ME. Incidence of myocarditis in peripartum cardiomyopathy. Am J Cardiol 1994; 74: 474–77.

[12] Midei MG, DeMent SH, Feldman AM, Hutchins GM, Baughman KL. Peripartum myocarditis and cardiomyopathy. Circulation 1990; 81: 922–28.

[13] Felker GM, Thompson RE, Hare JM, et al. Underlying causes and long-term survival in patients with initially unexplained cardiomyopathy. N Engl J Med 2000; 342:1077–84.

[14] Bultmann BD, Klingel K, Nabauer M, Wallwiener D, Kandolf R. High prevalence of viral genomes and inflammation in peripartum cardiomyopathy. Am J Obstet Gynecol 2005; 193:363–65.

[15] Pearson GD, Veille JC, Rahimtoola S, et al. Peripartum cardiomyopathy: National Heart, Lung, and Blood Institute and Office of Rare Diseases (National Institutes of Health) workshop recommendations and review. JAMA 2000;283:1183–88.

[16] Farber PA, Glasgow LA. Viral myocarditis during pregnancy: encephalomyocarditis virus infection in mice. Am Heart J 1970;80: 96–102.

[17] Lyden DC, Huber SA. Aggravation of coxsackievirus, group B, type 3-induced myocarditis and increase in cellular immunity to myocyte antigens in pregnant Balb/c mice and animals treated with progesterone. Cell Immunol 1984;87:462–72.

[18] O'Connell JB, Costanzo-Nordin MR, Subramanian R, et al. Peripartum cardiomyopathy: clinical, hemodynamic, histologic, and prognostic characteristics. J Am Coll Cardiol 1986;8:52–56.

[19] Kovithavongs T, Dossetor JB. Suppressor cells in human pregnancy. Transplant Proc 1978;10:911–3.

[20] Thong YH, Steele RW, Vincent MM, Hensen SA, Bellanti JA. Impaired in vitro cell-mediated immunity to rubella virus during pregnancy. N Engl J Med 1973;289:604–06.

[21] D'Cruz IA, Balani SG & Iyer LS. Infectious hepatitis and pregnancy. Obstet Gynecol 1968;31:449–55.

[22] Oakley, CM. Myocarditis, pericarditis and other pericardial diseases. Heart 2000;84:449–54.

[23] Coyne CB, Bergelson JM. Virus-induced Abl and Fyn kinase signals permit coxsackie virus entry through epithelial tight junctions. Cell 2006; 124: 119-31.

[24] Cooper LT, Rader V, Ralston NV. The roles of selenium and mercury in the pathogenesis of viral cardiomyopathy. Congest Heart Fail 2007; 13: 193-99.

[25] Mahfoud F, Gärtner B, Kindermann M, et al. Virus serology in patients with suspected myocarditis: utility or futility? Eur Heart J 2011; 32: 897-903.

[26] Murphy JG. Peripartum cardiomyopathy. In: Cooper LT, editor. Myocarditis: from bench to bedside. Totowa (NJ): Humana Press; 2003. p. 589–608.

[27] Bachmaier K, Neu N, de la Maza LM, Pal S, Hessel A, Penninger JM. Chlamydia infections and heart disease linked through antigenic mimicry. Science 1999;283:1335–39.

[28] Cenac A, Djibo A, Sueur JM, Chaigneau C, Orfila J. Chlamydia infection and peripartum dilated cardiomyopathy in Niger. Med Trop(Mars) 2000;60:137–40.

[29] Ansari AA, Neckelmann N, Wang YC, Gravanis MB, Sell KW, Herskowitz A. Immunologic dialogue between cardiac myocytes, endothelial cells and mononuclear cells. Clin Immunol Immunopathol 1993;68:208–14.

[30] Sliwa K, Skudicky D, Bergemann A, Candy G, Puren A, Sareli P. Peripartum cardiomyopathy: analysis of clinical outcome, left ventricular function, plasma levels of cytokines and Fas/APO-1. J Am Coll Cardiol 2000;35:701–05.

[31] Karaye KM, Henein MY Peripartum cardiomyopathy: A review article Int J C International Journal of Cardiology 2011;150:325-31.

[32] Ansari AA, Fett JD, Carraway RE, Mayne AE, Onlamoon N, Sundstrom JB. Autoimmune mechanisms as the basis for human peripartum cardiomyopathy. Clin Rev Allergy Immunol 2002; 23:301–324.

[33] Knobel B, Melamud E, Kishon Y. Peripartum cardiomyopathy. Isr J Med Sci 1984;20:1061–63.

[34] Ukena C, Mahfoud F, Kindermann I, et al. Prognostic electrocardiographic parameters in patients with suspected myocarditis. Eur J of Heart Failure 2011; 13: 398-405.

[35] Smith SC, Ladenson JH, Mason JW, et al. Elevations of cardiac troponin I associated with myocarditis. Experimental and clinical correlations. Circulation 1997;95:163–68.

[36] Forster O, Hilfiker-Kleiner D, Ansari AA, et al. Reversal of IFN-gamma, oxLDL and prolactin serum levels correlate with clinical improvement in patients with peripartum cardiomyopathy. Eur J Heart Fail 2008;10:861–68.

[37] Karjalainen J, Heikkila J. Incidence of three presentations of acute myocarditis in young men in military service: a 20 year experience. Eur Heart J 1999;20:1120–25.

[38] Galderisi M, Henein MY, D'hooge J, et al. European Association of Echocardiography. Recommendations of the European Association of Echocardiography: how to use echo-Doppler in clinical trials: different modalities for different purposes. Eur J Echocardiogr 2011;12:339–53.

[39] Mouquet F, Lions C, de Groote P, Bouabdallaoui N, Willoteaux S, Dagorn J, Deruelle P, Lamblin N, Bauters C, Beregi JP. Characterisation of peripartum cardiomyopathy by cardiac magnetic resonance imaging. Eur Radiol 2008;18: 2765–69.

[40] Di Bella G, de Gregorio C, Minutoli F, et al. Early diagnosis of focal myocarditis by cardiac magnetic resonance. Int J Cardiol 2007; 117:280–81.

[41] Baccouche H, Mahrholdt H, Meinhardt G, et al. Diagnostic synergy of non-invasive cardiovascular magnetic resonance and invasive endomyocardial biopsy in troponin-positive patients without coronary artery disease. Eur Heart J 2009; 30: 2869-79.

[42] De Wilde JP, Rivers AW, Price DL. A review of the current use of magnetic resonance imaging in pregnancy and safety implications for the fetus. Prog Biophys Mol Biol 2005;87:335–53.

[43] Laissy JP, Hyafil F, Feldman LJ, et al. Differentiating acute myocardial infarction from myocarditis: diagnostic value of early- and delayed-perfusion cardiac MR imaging. Radiology 2005; 237:75–82.

[44] Kanal E, Barkovich AJ, Bell C, et al. ACR guidance document for safe MR practices: 2007. AJR Am J Roentgenol 2007;188:1447–74.

[45] Webb JA, Thomsen HS, Morcos SK. The use of iodinated and gadolinium contrast media during pregnancy and lactation. Eur Radiol 2005;15:1234–40.

[46] Aretz HT, Billingham ME, Edwards WD. Myocarditis: a histopathological definition and classification. Am J Cardiovasc Pathol 1987;1:3–14.

[47] Lieberman EB, Hutchis GM, Herskowitz A, Rose NR, Baughman KL. Clinicopathologic description of myocarditis. J Am Coll Cardiol. 1991;18:1617-26.

[48] Leurent G, Baruteau AE, Larralde A, et al. Contribution of cardiac MRI in the comprehension of peripartum cardiomyopathy pathogenesis. Int J Cardiol 2009; 132:91–3.

[49] Cooper LT, Baughman KL, Feldman AM, et al. The role of endomyocardial biopsy in the management of cardiovascular disease: a scientific statement from the American Heart Association, the American College of Cardiology, and the European Society of Cardiology. Endorsed by the Heart Failure Society of America and the Heart Failure Association of the European Society of Cardiology. Eur Heart J 2007; 28:3076–93.

[50] Baughman KL. Peripartum cardiomyopathy. Curr Treat Options Cardiovasc Med 2001; 3:469–80.

[51] Vera Regitz-Zagrosek, Carina Blomstrom Lundqvist, Claudio Borghi et al. Guidelines on the management of cardiovascular diseases during pregnancy. The Task Force on the Management of Cardiovascular Diseases during Pregnancy of the European Society of Cardiology (ESC). Eur Heart J 2011; 32: 3147–97.

[52] John J.V. McMurray JJV, Adamopoulos S, Stefan D. Anker SD, et al. ESC Guidelines for the diagnosis and treatment of acute and chronic heart failure 2012. The Task Force for the Diagnosis and Treatment of Acute and Chronic Heart Failure 2012 of the European Society of Cardiology. Developed in collaboration with the Heart Failure Association (HFA) of the ESC. Eur Heart J 2012; 33: 1787–1847.

[53] Cooper WO, Hernandez-Diaz S, Arbogast PG, Dudley JA, Dyer S, Gideon PS, Hall K, Ray WA. Major congenital malformations after first-trimester exposure to ACE inhibitors. N Engl J Med 2006;354:2443–51.

[54] Andrade SE, Raebel MA, Brown J, et al. Outpatient use of cardiovascular drugs during pregnancy. Pharmacoepidemiol Drug Saf 2008; 17:240–47.

[55] Sliwa K, Fett J, Elkayam U. Peripartum cardiomyopathy. Lancet 2006; 368:687–93.

[56] Narin C, Reyhanoglu H, Tulek B, et al. Comparison of different dose regimens of enoxaparin in deep vein thrombosis therapy in pregnancy. Adv Ther 2008; 25:585–94.

[57] Khul U, Pauschinger M, Schwimmbeck PL, et al. Interferon-beta treatment eliminates cardiotropic viruses and improves left ventricular function in patients with myocardial persistence of viral genomes and left ventricular dysfunction. Circulation 2003; 107: 2793-98.

[58] Schmidt-Lucke C, Spillmann F, Bock T, et al. Interferon-beta modulates endothelial damage in patients with cardiac persistence of parvovirus B19V. J Infect Dis 2010; 201: 936-45.

[59] Fett JD. Inflammation and virus in dilated cardiomyopathy as indicated by endomyocardial biopsy. Int J Cardiol (2006)., 112:125–26.

[60] Frustaci A, Russo M, Chimenti C. Randomized study on the efficacy of immunosuppressive therapy in patients with virus-negative inflammatory cardiomyopathy: the TIMIC study. Eur Heart J 2009; 30: 1995–2002.

[61] Lui PP, Schultheiss HP. Myocarditis. In: Braunwald E, Zipes DP, Libby P, (eds). The Text Book Of Cardiovascular Medicine - 8th edition. WB Saundres Company, Philadelphia – Toronto 2007; 1775-92.

[62] Bozkurt B, Villaneuva FS, Holubkov R, et al. Intravenous immune globulin in the therapy of peripartum cardiomyopathy. J Am Coll Cardiol 1999;34:177– 80.

[63] McNamara DM, Holubkov R, Starling RC, et al. Controlled trial of intravenous immune globulin in recent-onset dilated cardiomyopathy. Circulation 2001; 103:2254–59.

[64] Herda L.R., Trimpert C., Nauke U.; et al. Effects of immunoadsorption and subsequent immunoglobulin G substitution on cardiopulmonary exercise capacity in patients with dilated cardiomyopathy, Am Heart J 2010;159: 809-16.

[65] Bulut D., Scheeler M., Wichmann T., Borgel J., Miebach T., Mugge A.; Effect of protein A immunoadsorption on T cell activation in patients with inflammatory dilated cardiomyopathy, Clin Res Cardiol. 2010; 99:633-38.

[66] Wang QQ, Wang YL, Yuan HT et al. Immune tolerance to cardiac myosin induced by anti-CD4 monoclonal antibody in autoimmune myocarditis rats. J Clin Immunol. 2006; 26(3): 213-21.

Chapter 7

Myocarditis in Children Requiring Critical Care Transport

Jordan S. Rettig and Gerhard K. Wolf

Additional information is available at the end of the chapter

http://dx.doi.org/10.5772/56177

1. Introduction

Myocarditis is an uncommon but potentially life-threatening presentation in pediatric patients requiring critical care transport. Patients may present with malignant arrhythmias and hemodynamic collapse, and may require transport to a center offering extracorporeal life support. In this chapter we aim to provide a brief overview of pediatric myocarditis, with a particular focus on considerations for stabilization and transport in acute fulminant myocarditis. These considerations include intubation and ventilation, hemodynamic support, induction of anesthesia and pharmacological considerations for sedation, patient triage, and choice of an appropriate receiving center.

1.1. Etiology

Myocarditis is an acute inflammatory disease of the myocardium, classically characterized by myocyte necrosis [1], which leads to ventricular dysfunction. There are several possible causes of myocarditis including infectious (viral, bacterial, fungal, yeast, parasitic, and protozoan) and non-infectious (immune mediated reactions, toxins, and other disorders). In many cases there is no identified cause. Most cases of pediatric myocarditis with a known etiology are caused by infections, in particular by viral infections [2]- [4], however a viral etiology may be difficult to detect. In a recent autopsy series examining 28 cases of myocarditis, viral analysis was done in 25 cases and was only positive in 9 of those. [5]

2. Epidemiology and clinical presentation

It has been estimated that pediatric cardiomyopathy occurs in between 1.13 and 1.24 per 100,000 patients, and more than 14% of these patients likely have cardiomyopathy from an infectious cause. [6]- [8] Klugman et al identified 216 cases of pediatric myocarditis over a one-year period in 35 different children's hospitals, making up 0.05% of all patients seen. This group concluded that pediatric patients with myocarditis have considerable variability in their outcomes, use more intensive care unit (ICU) resources, and die more often than children with other diagnoses. [9] There is a broad range of clinical presentation ranging from asymptomatic to fulminant and symptoms are often non-specific. Some patients present with constitutional symptoms, and complaints of chest pain and fatigue are common. Additionally there may be large variability between presentations in different age groups. Patients with cardiac dysfunction may have syncope, heart failure, arrhythmias, or shock. [1] Fulminant myocarditis occurs in approximately 20–30% of all cases, and clinically presents with severe hemodynamic deterioration, cardiogenic shock, severe ventricular dysfunction, and possibly life-threatening arrhythmias. [10] Unlike adult patients, children more commonly present with fulminant myocarditis. [11] Myocarditis is a significant cause of sudden death and may result in the development of cardiomyopathy in some affected children. [12], [13]

3. Diagnosis

The diagnosis of myocarditis is often difficult. In one series of 31 cases of myocarditis in a pediatric emergency department, 57% of patients had been previously evaluated by a physician and diagnosed with pneumonia or asthma. [14] The less controversial diagnostic modalities include chest x-ray, electrocardiogram (EKG) and echocardiogram. Sinus tachycardia on EKG with low-voltage QRS complexes is described as a classic finding. Beyond that there may be a variety of changes seen on EKG, including widened QRS complexes, non-specific ST changes, axis deviation, and/or Q waves. Patients may also present with arrhythmias including ventricular tachycardia, supraventricular tachycardia, and varying degrees of heart block.

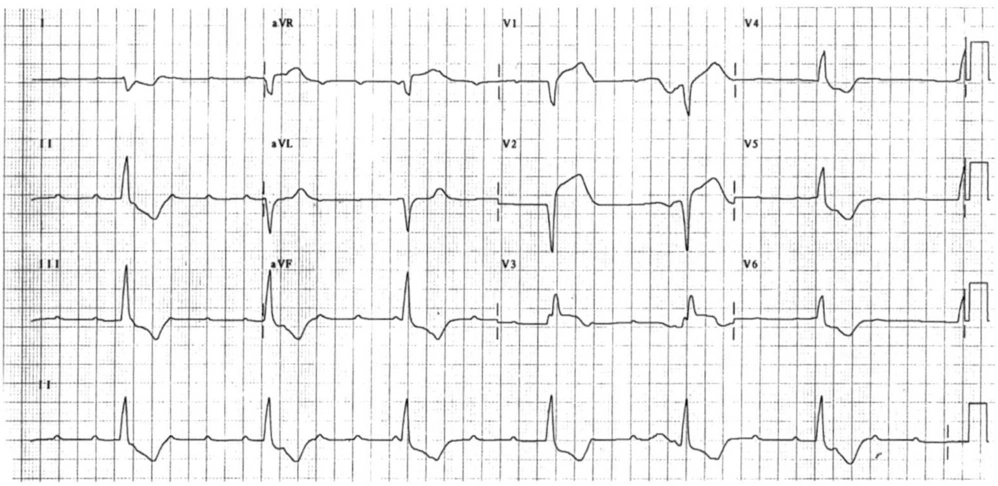

Figure 1. EKG of a 12 year old patient with myocarditis, atrioventricular block [15]

http://dx.doi.org/10.5772/56177

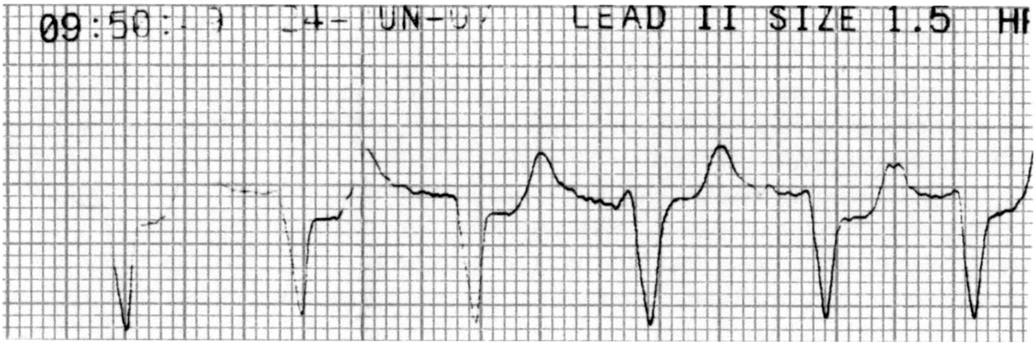

Figure 2. EKG (rhythm strip) of the same patient, who had ongoing severe ventricular dysfunction and developed intermittent episodes of wide-complex tachycardia [15]

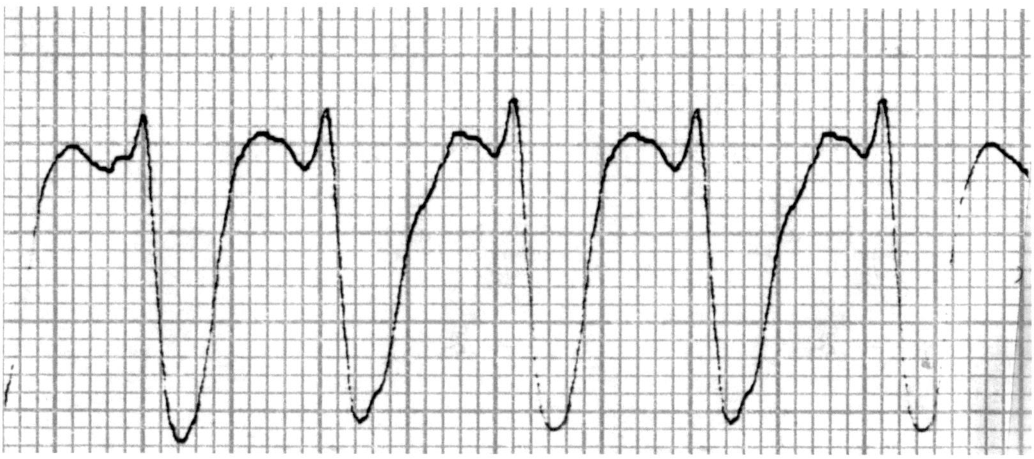

Figure 3. EKG (rhythm strip) of a 7 year old patient with myocarditis; wide-complex tachycardia [15]

Chest x-ray findings tend to be consistent with congestive heart failure, including cardiomegaly and increased pulmonary markings suggestive of pulmonary edema. Echocardiography is a useful adjunct to assess ventricular dimensions, function, and presence of atrioventricular valve regurgitation or pericardial effusion.

A recent review of diagnostic strategies for myocarditis concluded that enlarged ventricular dimensions on echocardiography and elevated cardiac troponin levels were the most common findings. [16] Troponin I has high specificity but limited sensitivity in the diagnosis of myocarditis, despite the fact that it is otherwise a reliable and commonly available biomarker of myocardial injury. [17] In children, cardiac troponin T has been reported to have a sensitivity of 71% in myocarditis. [18] Other common laboratory studies include general markers of inflammation or infection, such as complete blood count with differential, C-reactive protein and erythrocyte sedimentation rate. It is also useful to examine markers of end organ perfusion including lactate, liver function tests and creatinine. These studies may help understand the etiology and impact of the disease process, but none are specific for myocarditis.

More controversial diagnostic modalities include cardiac magnetic resonance (CMR) imaging and endomyocardial biopsy (EMB). In general these techniques would not be employed in an acute setting in a non-tertiary care center. CMR has the advantage of being non-invasive it requires specialty equipment and radiologists familiar with the interpretation of findings. EMB is controversial for a variety of reasons, especially since it is invasive and carries a risk of adverse events. Also, myocardial inflammation tends to be patchy and may be missed by biopsy. A recent consensus statement by the American College of Cardiology and the European Society of Cardiology made a class IIa recommendation for EMB in cases of unexplained cardiomyopathy in children. [19]

4. Transport considerations

4.1. Triage

Pediatric patients with symptomatic myocarditis should be admitted to a pediatric tertiary care center. Klugman et al. reported that in their cohort of pediatric myocarditis patients 45% of patients required milrinone, 35% needed epinephrine, and 25% were supported with mechanical ventilation. Extracorporeal membrane oxygenation was needed in 7% of patients, and cardiac transplantation in 5%. [9] When triaging the patient, consideration should be given to the fact that any patient requiring the use of blood pressure support in the setting of acute myocarditis may quickly deteriorate and need mechanical cardiovascular support. Extracorporeal membrane oxygenation (ECMO) support is now increasingly viewed as optimal supportive therapy in anticipation of full cardiac recovery. [20] In larger children, a ventricular assist device (VAD) has also been used to support ventricular function during acute illness. In a previously published paper reporting the transport a series of children with myocarditis, there were five out of ten patients who required ECMO. Among those five patients there were three survivors. [15] In another retrospective review of 36 cases of histologically confirmed myocarditis ECMO was used in 4 patients (11%). [21]

4.2. Transport

It has been estimated that fewer than ten percent of hospitals with intensive care unit beds have pediatric critical care beds. [22], [23] Therefore, pediatric admission to a tertiary intensive care unit frequently requires patient transport. Though emergency medical service teams are trained in basic pediatric resuscitation and stabilization, often times they do not have the breadth of experience or advanced training which would provide for the safest transport of the critically ill child. The use of a critical care transport teams on the other hand is strongly associated with decreased complication rates. [24]- [27] In particular for pediatric patients, the chance of an unplanned airway or cardiovascular event was 22 times greater when a critical care transport team was not used. [24] In any population of patients with a high risk for cardiopulmonary deterioration, consideration must be given to balancing the potential benefit of using a critical care transport team and the risk of holding the patient in the emergency department for a longer time period until the specialty team is available.

For the above reasons, patients who present with symptomatic myocarditis are best transported to a tertiary care center with a critical care transport team. These patients are at high risk for deteriorating during transport, and often require urgent interventions upon arrival at the receiving hospital. Helicopter transport may be faster than ground transport, although this is not always true in urban environments or if the involved facilities do not have an on-site helipad. [28] Helicopter transport guidelines have identified pediatric patients with symptomatic myocarditis as appropriate candidates for helicopter transport. [29] While an efficient mode of transport, medical helicopters have maximum distance limitations. There are also strict weather and altitude limitations to helicopter transport, which may affect ground and fixed wing transport to a lesser degree. A patient requiring frequent assessment or interventions may be challenging to care for in a helicopter due to noise, lack of space making access to the patient challenging and turbulence in flight. Additionally in a helicopter, and certainly in a fixed wing vehicle, it may be more difficult to divert to a different receiving facility should the patient become acutely unstable for transport. There is no evidence looking at pediatric myocarditis and ideal modes of transport. Data from adult patients shows that there are conflicting reports about the efficacy of different modes of transport, specifically helicopter versus ground transport. In 2012 a retrospective cohort study showed that among patients with major trauma admitted to level I or level II trauma centers, transport by helicopter compared with ground services was associated with improved survival to hospital discharge. [30] While there are earlier studies in agreement with these findings, other studies in the adult population have failed to show a benefit of helicopter transport. [31]- [34]

In summary, choosing a team and mode of transport for a patient is complex. There are many factors influencing decision-making surrounding patient transport. The medical team should consider the patient's anticipated medical needs and the risks of destabilization during transport, the urgency of the treatments needed at the receiving facility, transport logistics such as altitude, weather and distance, and the team availability and experience. [35]

4.3. Treatment

There are currently no specific therapies for acute fulminant myocarditis. The mainstay of therapy is supportive care to maintain cardiac output including mechanical ventilation, inotropic support and, if tolerated, afterload reduction and diuresis. For transport purposes intubation, ventilation and inotropic support play a larger role than other support strategies. In adult populations there have historically been more options for ventricular assist devices. However, pediatric assist devices have been successfully developed. In a recent study of the Excor Pediatric ventricular assist device (Berlin Heart), Fraser et al demonstrated that survival rates for patients awaiting heart transplant were significantly higher with the ventricular assist device than with ECMO. [36] This data is not specific for myocarditis, but is promising that assist devices can be effectively used in the pediatric population. Currently, the majority of patients with refractory cardiogenic shock and/or severe respiratory failure will likely require ECMO for ongoing support.

4.3.1. Intubation and sedation

In patients with evidence of pulmonary edema the risk of worsening hypoxemia and potential for respiratory acidosis is concerning, as neither would be well tolerated from a cardiac standpoint. As respiratory demands increase to compensate for these issues, the oxygen consumption of the respiratory muscles can increase up to eightfold. [37] Intubation and mechanical ventilation will reduce respiratory muscle oxygen consumption, and thus overall myocardial oxygen demand. [37] The risks of the induction for intubation should be carefully weighed against these benefits, but declining status may force a clinician to proceed with endotracheal intubation prior to transport.

In general, positive pressure ventilation reduces left ventricular wall tension and left ventricular afterload, and therefore may improve cardiac output by this mechanism. However, other cardiopulmonary interactions associated with intubation and positive pressure ventilation may precipitate low cardiac output or cardiac arrest in a patient with biventricular failure. Those potentially harmful interactions include cessation of right sided venous return during the transition from spontaneous breathing to positive pressure ventilation, and systemic vasodilation and negative inotropy induced by medication used for induction of anesthesia. If possible, it is important to ensure that the patient is euvolemic prior to induction to preserve right ventricular preload upon initiation of positive pressure ventilation. It is also advisable to have an inotropic agent either initiated or prepared to infuse to support biventricular function. [38]The choice of specific induction agents is less important than recognizing that patients in failure will likely have limited contractile reserve, will be relatively preload dependent and will not respond well to rapid changes in afterload. [39] The choice of the appropriate medication for induction of anesthesia for intubation is important. Any agent may precipitate vasodilation and cardiac depression. Etomidate is well-known for a low rate of adverse hemodynamic effects, and the direct sympathomimetic effects of ketamine may be particularly beneficial in shock states. [40] Carefully titrated low-dose fentanyl may also provide appropriate levels of sedation and analgesia with a more favorable cardiac profile. Midazolam, propofol, and barbiturates are all likely to trigger hypotension at induction doses and should therefore be avoided. Atropine premedication may be considered in pediatric patients with bradycardia, though many patients with myocarditis are tachycardic on presentation. [38]

The adverse hemodynamic effects of positive pressure ventilation on right sided venous return may be ameliorated by using a strategy to minimize mean airway pressure, thus reducing intrathoracic pressure. This includes avoiding lung hyperinflation, minimizing peak inspiratory pressures, the use of short inspiratory times and adequate expiratory times and conservative use of positive end-expiratory pressure (PEEP). While PEEP may be helpful in managing pulmonary edema and hypoxemia, it should be used with caution as it may lead to decreased right ventricular preload and increased right ventricular afterload.

4.3.2. Rate control

Both tachycardia and bradycardia can pose risks to a pediatric patient in acute heart failure. Arrhythmias must be quickly recognized and treated. Transcutaneous pacing has been recognized as an easy, safe, and effective temporary measure of rate control but may require sedation and likely requires analgesia in the pediatric patient. [41]- [44] As mentioned, administering sedation in a pediatric patient with myocarditis and cardiovascular compromise could lead to further hemodynamic instability. Initiation of catecholamines such as dopamine may provide benefit in patients with complete heart block by increasing the ventricular escape rate to improve systemic perfusion in transport and should be considered before initiation of transcutaneous pacing in hemodynamically stable patients. However, when using such agents care should be taken not to acutely increase left ventricular afterload.

4.3.3. Afterload reduction

Management of heart failure should be employed if the patient can tolerate diuresis and afterload reduction, but is probably not advisable in the acute setting. Ideally this management would include diuretics to lower filling pressures and angiotensin-converting enzyme (ACE) inhibitors to reduce systemic vascular resistance and left ventricular afterload. Beta-blockade may be used as well, however the only randomized controlled trial of beta-blockade for treatment of pediatric heart failure failed to demonstrate a benefit. [45] Furthermore using a beta-blocker in the acute setting may complicate resuscitation efforts should a patient have critically compromised output or lose circulation altogether. In patients with significant dysfunction and diminished cardiac output systemic inodilators such as milrinone, are often useful if tolerated. Due to the risk of systemic hypotension and some risk of worsening myocardial dysfunction these interventions are best started in a tertiary care setting, not during transport.

4.3.4. Levosimendan

Levosimendan is a positive ionotrope and functions by binding to cardiac troponin C to increase calcium sensitivity of myocytes. It also has vasodilatory effects in arterial, venous and coronary vasculature, which leads to afterload reduction and better matching of myocardial oxygen demand. [46]- [49] Therefore despite improving ventricular function, levosimendan does not significantly increase myocardial oxygen demand. Levosimendan is currently not FDA approved, so there is no collective experience with it the US centers. There are case reports of levosimendan being used successfully in both adult and pediatric myocarditis. [50]- [52] However, there are no larger, prospective studies to provide adequate evidence for routine use at this point. It remains unclear what potential benefit this drug would have in critical care transport.

4.3.5. IVIG

The benefit of immune modulation remains controversial, and is not usually an adjunct to consider during acute transport management. Intravenous immunoglobulins (IVIG) are the most commonly used immune modulator in myocarditis. Drucker et al. showed a statistically significant improvement in survival in pediatric patients treated with IVIG. [53] However McNamara conducted a randomized control trial in adults and failed to show any difference in survival among those treated with IVIG. [54] The data on the use of immunosuppressive agents such as prednisone, azathioprine and cyclosporine is not yet convincing. When the existing data was examined in a meta-analysis, Hia et al were not able to find statistical significance for improved outcomes. [55] That said, many centers currently use IVIG in the treatment of myocarditis and in certain cases immunosuppressive therapy may improve outcomes. [9], [56]

4.3.6. Mechanical support

In severe cases of cardiogenic shock patients may require rescue with veno-arterial (VA) ECMO or ventricular assist devices (VADs). Veno-venous (VV) ECMO is typically reserved for patients with predominant pulmonary failure. Whether requiring ECMO or VAD support, patients are best cared for in tertiary care centers with established ECMO programs.

VA-ECMO should be considered in patients with myocarditis only once routine supportive therapies have failed. [57], [58] While potentially life-sustaining in these cases, ECMO is not without risk. There is significant chance for hemorrhage, infectious complications and vascular injury during cannulation. There is also a risk of cerebral and coronary hypoxia and stroke. Less common, but potentially life-threatening are thrombotic events. Another complicating issue, which may ultimately compromise ventricular recovery, is left atrial hypertension secondary to poor ventricular function and decreased ejection while on ECMO. Left atrial hypertension can result in increased left ventricular end-diastolic pressure, subendocardial ischemia and pulmonary edema. There is no consensus on indications or technique for left atrial decompression, but it has been shown to relieve pulmonary edema and improve hemodynamics in one study. [59]

In experienced centers, ECMO is often successfully employed as a short-term rescue therapy for refractory cardiopulmonary failure. Though there is extensive experience with pediatric ECMO, in addition to potential complications there are also other significant limitations: need for sedation, lack of mobility, and relatively short lifespan of the circuit. In cases where failure is more chronic, or transplant is needed, a VAD may be a more appropriate intervention. VADs are available as right (RVAD), left (LVAD) and bi-ventricular (BiVAD) devices. They have been used for ventricular recovery, destination devices and as bridges to heart transplant. A recent prospective, single-group pediatric trial showed that survival rates to transplant were significantly higher with the ventricular assist device than with ECMO. [36] Complications of assist devices are significant and similar to ECMO, including bleeding, stroke, infection and thrombotic events.

4.3.7. Special consideration: ECMO on transport

Pediatric ECMO is offered in many centers worldwide [60], and increasingly ECMO centers are confronted with the request to transport a patient on ECMO. A few centers in the United States and in Europe reported these transports in the literature. [61]- [67] One group reported the successful transport of 68 children on ECMO, traveling a distance between eight and 7500 miles. Overall ECMO survival was comparable with in-house survival on

ECMO at the same institution. More importantly, no deaths occurred during ECMO transport. [66]

Bringing an ECMO team to a referring facility to place an unstable patient on extracorporeal support and then transport the patient back to a tertiary care center on ECMO has been suggested and, in a few cases, successfully completed. The logistics of providing such a service are very complicated. Based on military data, Coppola and colleagues reported that the ECMO transport team consists of 10-15 staff members, including a mission commander, a pediatric intensivist, a pediatric cardiologist, a pediatric surgeon, two to three ECMO specialists, nurses and respiratory therapists [66]. A civilian team reported using a team consisting of two nurses, two ECLS specialists, an attending physician, and a resident. [67] ECMO transports to date have been completed in ground, fixed-wing, and rotor-wing vehicles. The complexity of ECMO transport warrants careful discussion about feasibility and resource utilization, but may be successfully accomplished. That said, early referral to an ECMO center while the patient may be safely transported without ECMO is the preferred option.

5. Conclusions

Myocarditis presents with a broad range of relatively non-specific symptoms and for that reason is difficult to diagnose, but must remain on the list of differential diagnoses for any child presenting with acute heart failure or other signs of cardiac deterioration. Acute fulminant myocarditis is life-threatening and requires careful, proactive management. When treating the pediatric patient with acute fulminant myocarditis clinicians should consider the benefits of intubation, inotropic infusions, and transcutaneous pacing as temporizing measures especially during the transport phase, recognizing that any of those interventions can lead to further deterioration of the patient if not performed with great caution. Prompt and safe transport to a pediatric tertiary care center should be ensured. The option of early management with ECMO or other assist devices seems beneficial and should be considered when making triage decisions.

Author details

Jordan S. Rettig[1] and Gerhard K. Wolf[2*]

*Address all correspondence to: gerhard.wolf@childrens.harvard.edu

1 Division of Cardiac Critical Care, Department of Cardiology, Perioperative and Pain Medicine, Boston Children's Hospital, Harvard Medical School, Boston, Massachusetts, USA

2 Division of Critical Care Medicine, Department of Anesthesiology, Perioperative and Pain Medicine, Boston Children's Hospital, Harvard Medical School, Boston, Massachusetts, USA

References

[1] Liu, R, & Schulteiss, H. Myocarditis. In: Libby P, DL M, O'Bonow R, DP Z, eds. Brunwald's Heart Disease: A Textbook of Cardiovascular Medicine. 8th ed. Philadelphia: Saunders Elsevier; (2007)., 2007, 1775-85.

[2] Kearney, M. T, Cotton, J. M, Richardson, P. J, & Shah, A. M. Viral myocarditis and dilated cardiomyopathy: mechanisms, manifestations, and management. Postgrad Med J (2001)., 77, 4-10.

[3] Vashist, S, & Singh, G. K. Acute myocarditis in children: current concepts and management. Curr Treat Options Cardiovasc Med (2009)., 11, 383-91.

[4] Robinson, J, Hartling, L, Vandermeer, B, Crumley, E, & Klassen, T. P. Intravenous immunoglobulin for presumed viral myocarditis in children and adults. Cochrane Database Syst Rev (2005). CD004370.

[5] Weber, M. A, Ashworth, M. T, Risdon, R. A, Malone, M, Burch, M, & Sebire, N. J. Clinicopathological features of paediatric deaths due to myocarditis: an autopsy series. Arch Dis Child (2008)., 93, 594-8.

[6] Shekerdemian, L, & Bohn, D. Acute viral myocarditis: Epidemiology and pathophysiology.. Pediatr Crit Care Med (2006). SS7., 2.

[7] Sugent, A, & Daunbeney, P. P C. The epidemiology of childhood cardiomyopathy in Australia. N Engl J Med (2003)., 348, 1639-46.

[8] Lipshultz, S, Sleeper, L, & Towbin, J. The incidence of pediatric cardiomyopathy in two regions of the United States. N Engl J Med (2003)., 348, 1647-55.

[9] Klugman, D, Berger, J. T, Sable, C. A, He, J, Khandelwal, S. G, & Slonim, A. D. Pediatric patients hospitalized with myocarditis: a multi-institutional analysis. Pediatr Cardiol (2010)., 31, 222-8.

[10] Lieberman, E. B, Hutchins, G. M, Herskowitz, A, Rose, N. R, & Baughman, K. L. Clinicopathologic description of myocarditis. J Am Coll Cardiol (1991)., 18, 1617-26.

[11] Amabile, N, Fraisse, A, Bouvenot, J, Chetaille, P, & Ovaert, C. Outcome of acute fulminant myocarditis in children. Heart (2006)., 92, 1269-73.

[12] (Maron BJ, Doerer JJ, Haas TS, Tierney DM, Mueller FO. Sudden deaths in young competitive athletes: analysis of 1866 deaths in the United States, 1980-2006. Circulation 2009;119:1085-92). 119, 1085-92.

[13] Nugent, A. W, Daubeney, P. E, Chondros, P, et al. The epidemiology of childhood cardiomyopathy in Australia. N Engl J Med (2003)., 348, 1639-46.

[14] Freedman, S. B, Haladyn, J. K, Floh, A, Kirsh, J. A, Taylor, G, & Thull-freedman, J. Pediatric myocarditis: emergency department clinical findings and diagnostic evaluation. Pediatrics (2007). , 120, 1278-85.

[15] Wolf, G. K, Frakes, M. A, Gallagher, M, Allan, C. K, & Wedel, S. K. Management of suspected myocarditis during critical-care transport. Pediatr Emerg Care (2010). , 26, 512-7.

[16] Checchia, P, & Kulik, T. Acute viral myocarditis. Pediatr Crit Care Med (2006). SS11., 8.

[17] Smith, S. C, Ladenson, J. H, Mason, J. W, & Jaffe, A. S. Elevations of cardiac troponin I associated with myocarditis. Experimental and clinical correlates. Circulation (1997). , 95, 163-8.

[18] Soongswang, J, Durongpisitkul, K, Nana, A, et al. Cardiac troponin T: a marker in the diagnosis of acute myocarditis in children. Pediatr Cardiol (2005). , 26, 45-9.

[19] Cooper, L. T, Baughman, K. L, Feldman, A. M, et al. The role of endomyocardial biopsy in the management of cardiovascular disease: a scientific statement from the American Heart Association, the American College of Cardiology, and the European Society of Cardiology. Circulation (2007). , 116, 2216-33.

[20] Bohn, D, Macrae, D, & Chang, A. Acute viral myocarditis: mechanical circulatory support. Pediatr Crit Care Med (2006). SS4., 21.

[21] Lee, K. J, Mccrindle, B. W, Bohn, D. J, et al. Clinical outcomes of acute myocarditis in childhood. Heart (1999). , 82, 226-33.

[22] Randolph, A, Gonzales, C, Crotellini, L, & Yeh, T. Growth of pediatric intensive care units in the United States. Pediatrics (2004). , 144, 792-8.

[23] Guss, C, Brower, R, & Hudson, L. Indcidence of acute lung injury in the United States. Crit Care Med (2003). , 31, 1607-11.

[24] Orr, R. Unplanned events in pediatric critical care transport. Pediatrics (1999). S687.

[25] Edge, W, Kanter, R, & Weigle, C. Reduction of morbidity in interhospital transport by specialized pediatric staff. Crit Care Med (1994). , 22, 1186-91.

[26] Frakes, M. Flight team management of in-place endotracheal tubes. Air Med J (2002). , 21, 29-31.

[27] Gebermichael, M. Interhospital transport of the extremely ill patient. Crit Care Med (2000). , 28, 79-85.

[28] Svenson, J, Connor, O, & Lindsay, J. B. A comparison of air versus ground transport times for interfacility transfers in a regional referral system. Air Med J (2005). , 24, 70-2.

[29] Thompson, D, & Thomas, S. Guidelines for air medical dispatch. Prehosp Emerg Care (2003). , 7, 265-71.

[30] Galvagno, S. M. Jr., Haut ER, Zafar SN, et al. Association between helicopter vs ground emergency medical services and survival for adults with major trauma. JAMA (2012). , 307, 1602-10.

[31] Rose, M. K, Cummings, G. R, Rodning, C. B, Brevard, S. B, & Gonzalez, R. P. Is helicopter evacuation effective in rural trauma transport? Am Surg (2012). , 78, 794-7.

[32] Shepherd, M. V, Trethewy, C. E, Kennedy, J, & Davis, L. Helicopter use in rural trauma. Emerg Med Australas (2008). , 20, 494-9.

[33] Stewart, K. E, Cowan, L. D, Thompson, D. M, Sacra, J. C, & Albrecht, R. Association of direct helicopter versus ground transport and in-hospital mortality in trauma patients: a propensity score analysis. Acad Emerg Med (2011). , 18, 1208-16.

[34] Butler, D. P, Anwar, I, & Willett, K. Is it the H or the EMS in HEMS that has an impact on trauma patient mortality? A systematic review of the evidence. Emerg Med J (2010). , 27, 692-701.

[35] Blumen, I, Corbett, P, & Krost, W. Considerations in vehicle selection for patient transport. In: Blumen I, ed. Principles and direction of air medical transport. Salt Lake City: Air Medical Physician's Association; (2006).

[36] Fraser, C. D. Jr., Jaquiss RD, Rosenthal DN, et al. Prospective trial of a pediatric ventricular assist device. N Engl J Med (2012). , 367, 532-41.

[37] Mason, R, Murray, E, Broaddus, V, & Nadel, J. Murray and Nadel's Textbook of Respiratory Medicine. 4th ed. Philadelphia: Saunders; (2005).

[38] Miller, R. Anesthesia. 6th ed. New York: Churchill Livingstone; (2005).

[39] DiNardo JAZvara DA. Anesthesia for cardiac surgery. 3rd ed. Malden, Mass.: Blackwell Pub.; (2008).

[40] Bergen, J, & Smith, D. A review of etomidate for rapid sequence intubation in the emergency department. J Emerg Med (1997). , 15, 221-30.

[41] Altamaura, G, & Toscano, S. LoBianco F, Catalno F, Pistolese M. Emergency cardiac pacing for severe bradycardia. Pacing Clin Electrophysiol (1990). , 13, 2038-43.

[42] Madsen, J, Meiborn, J, Videbak, R, Pedersen, F, & Grande, P. Transcutaneous pacing: Experience with the Zoll noninvasive temporary pacemaker. Am Heart J (1988). , 116, 7-10.

[43] Zoll, P, & Zoll, R. Noninvasive temporary cardiac stimulation. Crit Care Med (1985). , 13, 925-6.

[44] Belano, M, Hesslein, P, Finlay, C, Faerron-angel, J, Williams, W, & Rowe, R. Noninvasive transcutaneous pacing in children. Pacing Clin Electrophysiol (1987). , 10, 1262-70.

[45] Shaddy, R. E, Boucek, M. M, Hsu, D. T, et al. Carvedilol for children and adolescents with heart failure: a randomized controlled trial. JAMA (2007). , 298, 1171-9.

[46] Parissis, J. T, Adamopoulos, S, Antoniades, C, et al. Effects of levosimendan on circulating pro-inflammatory cytokines and soluble apoptosis mediators in patients with decompensated advanced heart failure. Am J Cardiol (2004). , 93, 1309-12.

[47] Parissis, J. T, & Filippatos, G. Levosimendan in viral myocarditis: not only an inodilator but also a cardioprotector? Eur J Clin Invest (2009). , 39, 839-40.

[48] Pollesello, P, & Papp, Z. The cardioprotective effects of levosimendan: preclinical and clinical evidence. J Cardiovasc Pharmacol (2007). , 50, 257-63.

[49] Antila, S, Sundberg, S, & Lehtonen, L. A. Clinical pharmacology of levosimendan. Clin Pharmacokinet (2007). , 46, 535-52.

[50] Schweigmann, U, Velik-salchner, C, Kilo, J, & Schermer, E. How mechanical circulatory support helps not to need it--new strategies in pediatric heart failure. Artif Organs (2011). , 35, 1105-9.

[51] Busani, S, Pasetto, A, Ligabue, G, Malavasi, V, Lugli, R, & Girardis, M. Levosimendan in a case of severe peri-myocarditis associated with influenza A/H1N1 virus. Br J Anaesth (2012). , 109, 1011-3.

[52] Latva-hirvela, J, Kyto, V, Saraste, A, Vuorinen, T, Levijoki, J, & Saukko, P. Effects of levosimendan in experimental acute coxsackievirus myocarditis. Eur J Clin Invest (2009). , 39, 876-82.

[53] Drucker, N. A, Colan, S. D, Lewis, A. B, et al. Gamma-globulin treatment of acute myocarditis in the pediatric population. Circulation (1994). , 89, 252-7.

[54] Mcnamara, D. M, Holubkov, R, Starling, R. C, et al. Controlled trial of intravenous immune globulin in recent-onset dilated cardiomyopathy. Circulation (2001). , 103, 2254-9.

[55] Hia, C. P, Yip, W. C, Tai, B. C, & Quek, S. C. Immunosuppressive therapy in acute myocarditis: an 18 year systematic review. Arch Dis Child (2004). , 89, 580-4.

[56] Camargo, P. R, & Snitcowsky, R. da Luz PL, et al. Favorable effects of immunosuppressive therapy in children with dilated cardiomyopathy and active myocarditis. Pediatr Cardiol (1995). , 16, 61-8.

[57] Chen, Y. S, Wang, M. J, Chou, N. K, et al. Rescue for acute myocarditis with shock by extracorporeal membrane oxygenation. Ann Thorac Surg (1999). , 68, 2220-4.

[58] Duncan, B. W, Bohn, D. J, Atz, A. M, French, J. W, Laussen, P. C, & Wessel, D. L. Mechanical circulatory support for the treatment of children with acute fulminant myocarditis. J Thorac Cardiovasc Surg (2001). , 122, 440-8.

[59] Aiyagari, R. M, Rocchini, A. P, Remenapp, R. T, & Graziano, J. N. Decompression of the left atrium during extracorporeal membrane oxygenation using a transseptal cannula incorporated into the circuit. Crit Care Med (2006). , 34, 2603-6.

[60] The ELSO Registry(2009). Accessed 2009, at http://www.elso.med.umich.edu/Registry.htm.)

[61] Heulitt, M, Taylor, B, & Faulkner, S. Interhospital transport of neonatal patients on extracorporeal membrane oxygenation: mobile-ECMO. Pediatrics (1995). , 95, 562-6.

[62] Rossaint, R, Pappert, D, & Gerlach, H. Extracorporeal membrane oxygenation for transport of hypoxemic patients with severe ARDS. Br J Anesth (1997). , 78, 241-6.

[63] Linden, V, Palmer, K, & Reinhard, J. Interhospital transportation of patients with severe acute respiratory failure on extracorporeal membrane oxygenation- national and international experience. Intensive Care Med (2001). , 27, 1643-8.

[64] Foley, D, Pranikoff, T, & Younger, J. A review of 100 patients transported on extracorporeal life support. ASAIO J (2002). , 48, 612-9.

[65] Huang, S, Chen, Y, & Chi, N. Out-of-center extracorporeal membrane oxygenation for adult cardiogenic shock patients. Artif Organs (2006). , 30, 24-8.

[66] Coppola, C, Tyree, M, & Larry, K. DiGeronimo R. A 22-year experience in global transport extracorporeal membrane oxygenation. J Pediatr Surg (2008). , 43, 46-52.

[67] Bowers, W, & Wyrick, P. Extracorporeal life support: A transcontinental transport experience. Air Med J (2003). , 12, 7-11.

Section 5

Treatment

Chapter 8

New Trends in the Development of Treatments of Viral Myocarditis

Decheng Yang, Huifang Mary Zhang, Xin Ye,
Lixin Zhang and Huanqin Dai

Additional information is available at the end of the chapter

http://dx.doi.org/10.5772/54103

1. Introduction

Viral myocarditis is caused by a variety of viruses of more than 10 genera, such as coxsackievirus, adenovirus, parvovirus, hepatitis c virus, herpes virus, influenza virus, HIV, etc. [1]. However, the most frequently reported and extensively studied one is coxsackievirus B3 (CVB3), which causes ~30% of all viral myocarditis cases [2]. Thus, in this chapter the review will mainly focus on CVB3-induced myocarditis. This virus can infect multiple organs of human such as heart, pancreas, brain, liver, lung, spleen, etc. and cause myocarditis, pancreatitis, meningitis, hepatitis, etc. However, the most fatal disease is myocarditis, particular in children and young people [3]. Viral myocarditis is characterized by inflammatory infiltration of immune cells in the heart muscle after viral infection. This viral infection can cause direct damage of cardiomyocytes as well as immune-mediated destructions of the myocardium, leading to cardiac dysfunction. In addition, viral myocarditis often progresses into dilated cardiomyopathy (DCM), an end-stage heart dysfunction. Patients with DCM usually require heart transplantation [4]. There is no other treatment option at the present. Viral myocarditis is one of the major life-threatening diseases in children. It is the cause of ~ 20% of sudden unexpected death in young people [5]. To date, there is no specific treatment for this viral infection.

CVB3 is a positive single-stranded, non-enveloped RNA virus of the enterovirus genus of the *Picornaviridae* family. Its genome is ~7.4 kb long, containing a single long open reading frame (encoding 11 proteins) flanked by the 5′ and 3′ untranslated regions (UTRs). The 5′ UTR is 741 nucleotides (nt) long and harbors a number of cis-acting translational elements, such as the internal ribosomal entry site (IRES) and the cloverleaf sequence [6-9], which are crucial structures for viral translation and transcription. The 3′ UTR is a 99-nt long segment attached with a poly-A tail. The 3′ UTR folds to form kissing-loop tertiary structures, which are believed to play a role in facilitating viral transcription of the negative strand of CVB3 replication intermediate [10, 11]. The viral genomic RNA can directly serve as a mRNA template for translation of a single long polyprotein, which is processed by viral proteases to produce eleven individual proteins, among which four are structural proteins, VP1-VP4, and seven are non-structural proteins including proteases 2A and 3C, as well as a RNA-dependent RNA polymerase 3D. These three enzymatic proteins play important roles in viral life cycle and pathogenesis.

CVB3 infects cardiomyocytes by endocytosis through viral receptor CAR (coxsackie and adenovirus receptor) co-localized with tight junction proteins (e.g., occludin) [12]. It is also known that CAR-binding site (anti-receptor) on CVB3 particle lies in the canyon on the capsid surface. Upon attachment of CVB3 particles to CAR, the receptor changes conformation to form the viral A-particle, a product of the interactions between CVB3 and CAR, which then allows for the release of viral RNA into host cells and begins viral translation and transcription. The observation that soluble CAR protein can function as a virus trap leading to inactive A-particles has suggested a strategy for CVB3 therapy [13-15]. Depending on the different combination of viral strains and mouse models in the study of CVB3 infection, a CVB3 co-receptor called decay accelerating factor (DAF, CD55) is sometimes also necessary for CVB3 entry into the host cells [16, 17]. Thus, genes encoding CAR and DAF are important candidates for study of viral tropism and rational targets for antiviral drug design.

In recent years, extensive researches have been conducted for drug development. Although effective treatments are still not clinically available for this viral disease, some research strategies are very promising and have made exciting progresses. This chapter will first briefly summarize the current treatments used clinically for viral myocarditis even though they are not very specific and effective. Then we will focus on recent advances in new drug development, which include nucleic acid (NA)-based strategies, natural compounds, cell-based therapy, etc. We will also briefly discuss the limitations and challenges faced by the development of such treatments.

2. Current treatments

To date, there is no clinically proven specific treatment for viral myocarditis and DCM. Patients with DCM eventually need heart transplantation as the final option [18]. Managements for viral myocarditis are usually supportive therapies, such as improvements in hemodynamics with drugs used to treat other kinds of heart diseases, and application of non-specific antiviral agents to decrease viral load. The former include administration of angiotensin-converting enzyme inhibitors or angiotensin receptor blockade, beta-adrenergic blockade, diuretics, etc. [18-20]. The latter include application of type I interferon or nucleotide analogs such as ribavirin, which was reviewed elsewhere [3, 18, 19, 21, 22]. If it is caused by an autoimmune disorder, myocarditis would be appropriately treated by immunosuppression [18, 20]. However, the effectiveness of treatment with immunosuppressive therapies has not reached a consensus amongst different studies. This can probably be attributed to the difficulty of confirmation and diagnosis of the etiology and pathogenesis of myocarditis. Thus, it is very important to distinguish between infectious and autoimmune disease, since the same methods of treatment will not be optimal for both forms of heart muscle diseases. The diagnostic gold standard is endomyocardial biopsies with the histological Dallas criteria, in association with new immunohistochemical and viral PCR analyses of cardiac tissues [23]. In case of confirmed autoimmune-related disease and lack of detectable viral infection, an immunosuppressive treatment combining corticoids and azathioprine may be beneficial [24]. However, if the disease is primarily caused by viral infections, more specific antiviral agents would be the ideal drugs of choice.

In recent years, the search for such antiviral drugs has become a new trend in drug development for treatment of viral myocarditis. One of the strategies for developing such antivirals is the screening of chemical compounds, such as pleconaril, capable of interacting with picornavirus (particularly human rhinovirus) anti-receptor to block viral entry into the host cells [25-27]. Pleconaril functions in a mechanism similar to that of WIN compounds, by interacting with the hydrophobic amino acid residues located within the canyon floor of the anti-receptor of host cell. Thus, it results in the blockage of the attachment of viral particles to the host cell surface and reduces viral load in the heart [28]. Furthermore, the binding of WIN compounds also results in increased protein rigidity and stabilizes the entire viral capsid against enzymatic degradation, so that viral uncoating and release of viral RNA into the cytoplasm is inhibited [29, 30]. Pleconaril was initially developed for treatment of human common cold caused by human rhinovirus, a close relative of CVB3. It also shows effectiveness in inhibiting CVB3 infection [31]. To avoid mutation escape induced by pleconaril, new pleconaril derivatives have been synthesized and successfully tested against pleconaril-resistant mutants [32]. However, due to its high toxicity, pleconaril has not passed the approval by FDA of USA and is only used in a compassionate manner.

3. New strategies in drug development

3.1. Nucleic acid (NA)-based antivirals against CVB3 infection

3.1.1. Anti-CVB3 antisense oligonucleotides (ASONs)

ASONs are designed to bind to a complementary sequence in the target mRNA to form RNA-DNA heteroduplexes. These double-stranded hybrid sequences are recognized by RNase H, which digests the RNA strand in the duplex. Due to major problems, including instability, non-specific delivery, and unwanted side effects of the ASONs, the structure of this molecule has been modified extensively at different components (i.e., bases, sugar, or phosphate backbone), and has entered its third generation. The first generation of chemical modification was designed to enhance nuclease resistance of ASON in serum [33]. The representative of such is the phosphorothioate (PS) oligonucleotide (ON), in which one of the non-bridging oxygen atoms in the phosphodiester bond is replaced by sulfur, intended to prevent cleavage by nucleases. Early antiviral PS-modified ASONs exhibited the antisense properties of phosphodiester

ASONs, such as the ability to induce RNase H activation, while showing enhanced stability [34]. Another strategy to increase the stability of ASONs is the addition of alkyl groups at the 2 position of the ribose. 2-O-methyl (OMe) and 2-O-methoxy-ethyl (MOE) substitutions sterically shield the backbone from nuclease access, and also increase affinity to the target [35]. These modified ASONs function mainly by blocking translation via steric hindrance of elongating ribosome but not by RNAse H-mediated cleavage. In order to retain the advantage of the RNAse H mechanism, chimeric oligos containing both 2 unmodified and 2-modified DNAs, called gapmers, were conceived. The 2-O-alkyl modified ASONs and mixed backbone gapmer ASONs represent a second generation of ASON. The third generation ASONs are phosphorodiamidate morpholino oligonucleotides (PMOs). PMOs have a structure in which the ribose is replaced by a morpholine moiety and phosphorodiamidate (O-PONH2-O) linkers are used instead of phosphodiester bonds. Thus, PMOs are resistant to digestion by nucleases and are electrically neutral. PMO-RNA hybrids do not activate RNase H. Therefore, the mechanism by which PMOs inhibit protein synthesis is via binding the critical mRNA elements, such as the mRNA 5′UTR or the start codon region, to prevent ribosomes from binding or scanning.

CVB3, one of the most frequently used model systems for study of viral replication and pathogenesis, is also widely employed for evaluation of NA-based antiviral agents. The early investigations mainly focused on the application of the second and third generations of ASONs. McManus and coworkers are one of the pioneer groups to study the potential possibility to inhibit CVB3 replication using ASONs. Their earliest work using regular ASONs to target the different sites of 5′ UTR of CVB3 genome successfully mapped the IRES by *in vitro* translation inhibition assay [9]. That study provided useful information for the design of ASON for inhibiting CVB3 replication *in vitro* and in mouse models. Later, they used PS-ASONs targeting the 5′ and 3′ UTRs as well as the start codon region, and found that the oligomers targeting the 5′ and 3′ proximate ends of the CVB3 genome are the most effective candidates to inhibit viral replication in HeLa cells. Each of these two ASONs resulted in ~80% reduction of viral particle production, which is followed by the candidates targeting the IRES and the initiation codon region [36]. The importance of these sites for ASON binding was further confirmed by *in vivo* evaluation using a murine myocarditis model, although the antiviral efficiency is not as high as that obtained from *in vitro* evaluation [37].

To improve the stability of the oligomers, our group designed eight PMOs targeting both the sense and antisense strands of the CVB3 replication intermediate. To increase the efficiency of drug internalization, the PMOs were conjugated to a cell-penetrating arginine-rich peptide. These modified ASONs were evaluated in HeLa cells and HL-1 cardiomyocytes in culture and in a murine myocarditis model [38]. One of the oligomers, designed to target a sequence in the 3′ portion of the CVB3 IRES, was found to be especially potent against CVB3. Treatment of cells with this oligomer prior to CVB3 infection produced an approximately 3-log10 decrease in viral titer and largely protected cells from virus-induced cytopathic effect. A similar antiviral effect was observed when this oligomer treatment began shortly after the virus infection period. A/J mice receiving intravenous administration of this oligomer once prior to and once after CVB3 infection showed an ~2-log10-decreased viral titer in the myocardium at 7 days post infection and a significantly decreased level of cardiac tissue damage, compared to the controls [38].

In addition to the many ASON reports, another strategy using CpG containing oligodeoxynucleotide to activate antiviral immunity has been reported [39]. The mechanism is that the C-type of CpG oligomer can induce anti-CVB3 activity in human peripheral blood mononuclear cells through the induction of synthesis of natural mixed interferons.

3.1.2. *Antiviral ribozymes*

Ribozymes are catalytically active small RNA (~30-100 nts) molecules that act as enzymes to specifically cleave single strand RNA without the need of proteins. A major therapeutic advantage of ribozymes is the ability to make them trans-acting and to confer specificity to virtually cleave any target sequence [40]. This can be achieved by fusing the ribozyme core sequence at the 5′ and 3′ ends with the sequences that are complementary to the target sequence.

Ribozyme as an antiviral agent has been tested for many viral infections; however, report on anti-CVB3 has not been documented. Here, we will take HCV as an example to briefly discuss the potential application of ribozyme for the treatment of HCV infection, as many recent reports found that HCV is a new causal agent of myocarditis [41, 42]. To investigate the potential application of synthetic, stabilized ribozymes for the treatment of chronic HCV infection, Macejak et al. designed and synthesized hammerhead ribozymes targeting 15 conserved sites in the 5′ UTR of HCV RNA including the IRES [43]. It was shown that the inhibitory activity of ribozyme targeting site at nt 195 of HCV RNA exhibited a sequence-specific dose response, required an active catalytic ribozyme core, and was dependent on the presence of the HCV 5′ UTR. In an investigation of new genetic approaches on the management of this infection, six hammerhead ribozymes directed against a conserved region of the plus strand and minus strand of the HCV genome were isolated from a ribozyme library that was expressed using recombinant adenovirus vectors [44]. Treatment with synthetic stabilized anti-HCV ribozymes and vector-expressed HCV ribozymes has the potential to aid in treatment of patients who are infected with HCV by reducing the viral burden through specific targeting and cleavage of the viral genome. Gonzalez-Carmona and colleagues used RNA transcripts from a construct encoding a HCV-5'-NCR-luciferase fusion protein to test four chemically modified HCV specific ribozymes in a cell-free system and in HepG2 or CCL13 cell lines. They found that ribozyme (Rz1293) showed an inhibitory activity of viral translation of more than 70%, thus verifying that the GCA 348 cleavage site in the HCV loop IV is an accessible target site in cell culture and may be suitable for the development of novel optimized hammerhead structures [45].

3.1.3. *Anti-CVB3 siRNAs*

Accumulated evidence suggests that RNA interference (RNAi) plays an important role in the antiviral defense mechanism in mammalian cells [46-49]. These findings fueled the interests of researchers to use RNAi for antiviral drug development [49, 50].

The specificity of RNA silencing is mediated by small RNAs called short interfering RNAs (siRNA) and microRNA (miRNA). Both types of RNAs are generated by processing of ribonucleases in the Dicer family, a group of class III endoribonucleases, which cleaves double stranded non-coding RNA into fragments with a length of 21-25 nts. For siRNA, the long dsRNA or transgene-expressed short hairpin RNA (shRNA) are cleaved by Dicer. These RNAs are assembled into a multi-component complex, known as the RNA-induced silencing complex (RISC), which incorporates a single strand (antisense strand) of the siRNA serving as a guide sequence to silence the target gene [51, 52] (Figure. 1). For miRNA, this endogenous gene regulator is processed from primary miRNA (pri-miRNA) transcripts of non-coding regions or introns of protein-coding polymerase II transcripts. They are processed by RNase III Drosha to produce approximately 70-nt long pre-miRNAs, which are transported into cytoplasm by exportin-5 and are cleaved by Dicer to become the functional miRNA. Similar to siRNA, they also form a RISC with Argonaut proteins (having RNase H activity) and bind to their target mRNAs. The modes of actions of siRNA and miRNA depend on the degree of complementation between the siRNA or miRNA and their target sequences. siRNAs usually target coding regions by complementary base-paring and induce sequence-specific cleavage of mRNA substrate [53]; however, miRNAs preferentially recognize target sequences in the 3′ UTR of mRNAs and these target sites are often in multi-copy [54-57]. The binding of the miRNAs often takes place with an incomplete base-pairing, although a perfect base-pairing in the seed region (positions nt 2-8 from 5 end of the antisense strand) of miRNA forms the core of interaction. Depending on the complete or partial complementarities between the miRNA and mRNA, the outcome can be cleavage of the target mRNA or repression of translation (Figure. 1) [58, 59].

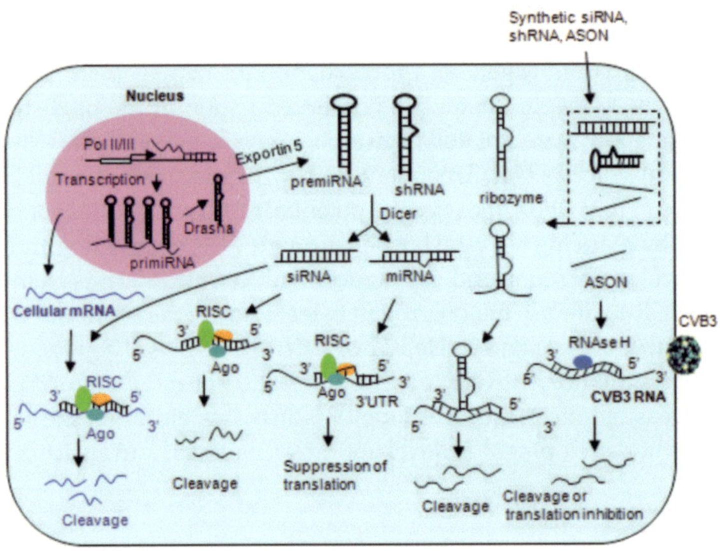

Figure 1. NA-based antiviral strategies to treat viral myocarditis. Antiviral nucleic acid molecules can either be transfected into cells or expressed intracellularly. ASONs hybridize to viral mRNA to induce RNase H-mediated cleavage of RNA strand of the DNA-RNA duplexes. Some modified ASONs cannot induce RNase H but they have a high affinity for the target and inhibit translation by steric hindrance of ribosome. Binding of ribozymes to the target sequence can trigger cleavage of the viral RNA. siRNAs incorporated in the RISC target the viral RNA by perfect sequence complementation and induce cleavage of the target sequence by RNAse H activity of Ago protein. miRNAs (or AmiRNAs) target viral RNA by imperfect sequence complementation and induce gene silencing by destabilizing mRNAs and suppression of translation. In addition, siRNAs can also target cellular genes (e.g., viral receptor and signal molecules) involved in viral entry and replication.

http://dx.doi.org/10.5772/54103

RNAi-mediated antiviral strategies can achieve much higher efficiency than ASONs. Thus, recent studies have focused on the design and evaluation of anti-CVB3 siRNAs. This group of small double-stranded RNAs, as a silencer of target gene expression, can virtually inhibit any genes of virus and cell if the site of targeting within the gene is unique. Thus, the target search for anti-CVB3 siRNAs is not only concentrating on CVB3 genome but also extending to the host cellular genes required for viral infection or replication.

3.1.3.1. Targeting the CVB3 genome

CVB3 genome harbors many cis-acting sequence elements for viral transcription and translation, such as the 5′ and 3′ UTRs, IRES, and other segments for binding of transcription and translation initiation factors. In addition, the viral genome also encodes many essential enzymes for CVB3 multiplication, such as proteases 2A and 3C as well as the RNA-dependent RNA polymerase 3D. These structures are rational targets for design of anti-CVB3 siRNAs. This hypothesis has been tested by a number of groups. The earlier selection of the siRNA targets was focused on CVB3 protease 2A. Almost at the same time, two groups independently found that inhibition of 2A protease by specific siRNAs significantly reduced CVB3 replication. Our laboratory evaluated five siRNAs targeting the 5′ UTR, AUG start codon, VP1, 2A and 3D, respectively and found that the siRNA targeting 2A (nts 3543-3561) showed strongest anti-CVB3 activity in HeLa cells, resulting in 92% reduction of viral replication and siRNAs targeting VP1, 3D and the 5′UTR showed modest antiviral effects, respectively. By mutational analysis of the mechanism of siRNA action, we further found that siRNA functions by targeting the positive strand of the virus and require a perfect sequence match in the central region of the target, but mismatches were more tolerated near the 3′ end than the 5′ end of the antisense strand [60]. This finding on the targeting of siRNA to positive strand of CVB3 was further supported by a later study using siRNA targeting the CVB3 3D gene [61]. We later also conjugated the siRNA-2A with folate to achieve specific delivery of the drug into HeLa cells and inhibited CVB3 replication[62].The second group that studied the siRNA targeting CVB3 2A by Merl and co-workers evaluated antiviral activity of siRNA-2A (nts 3637-3657) *in vitro* and in highly susceptible type I interferon receptor-knockout mice. They found that siRNA-2A led to a significant reduction of viral tissue titers, attenuated tissue injury and prolonged survival of mice [63]. It is very interesting to point out that although the two groups used different targeting sequences within the 2A RNA, they all achieved high efficiency of antiviral effects. However, the later work by Racchi et al., which used these two siRNAs together to transfect HeLa cells and then infect with CVB3 did not potentiate the anti-CVB3 effect compared with an equimolar concentration of either siRNA [64].

CVB3 RNA polymerase 3D is probably the most frequently used target for design of anti-CVB3 siRNAs as it is the only viral enzyme involved in CVB3 RNA replication. To date, at least a half dozen of studies on 3D have been reported. The earlier *in vitro* investigations used either un-modified or LNA-modified siRNAs or plasmid vector-expressed shRNAs and all achieved significant reduction of viral replication in CVB3-infected HeLa or Cos-7 cells [60, 61, 65-67]. The *in vivo* evaluation using mouse models also showed very promising results. One study employing transient transfection for *in vivo* mouse models demonstrated that two of the six candidate siRNAs targeting 3D and VP1, respectively, exerted strong anti-CVB3 effects in viral replication, accompanied by attenuated pancreatic tissue damage [68]. Another *in vivo* study is the intravenous treatment of mice with an adeno-associated virus vector (AAV2.9) expressing a shRNA targeting 3D [69]. Intravenous injection of recombinant AAV2.9 significantly attenuated cardiac dysfunction compared to vector-treated control mice on day 1 after CVB3 infection. Recently, a study by combination of soluble CAR receptor (sCAR-Fc) and siRNA targeting 3D achieved a synergistic effect in antiviral effect in human myocardial fibroblast cell culture [14].

Other less frequently used CVB3 target genes are protease 3C, structural protein VP1 and non-structural protein 2C. Like protease 2A, protease 3C also plays an important role in the viral life cycle by processing CVB3 polyproteins to generate mature individual structural and non-structural proteins after initial cleavage by 2A [70, 71]. One study designed three siRNAs targeting genes encoding 3C, 2A and 3D of CVB4. Evaluation by transfection of rhabdomyosarcoma (RD) cells demonstrated that siRNA-3C was the most potent siRNA among these three in inhibition of CVB4 replication. This antiviral activity was followed by siRNAs targeting 3D and 2A [72]. The difference in efficiency of these siRNAs was discussed by these authors and they proposed that this may be due to differences in function of these viral enzymes, which are encoded by these regions. The 3C region encodes a protease 3C which is responsible for the majority of cleavage of the viral polyprotein [71] and 3C as well as its precursor 3CD also plays an important role at the level of viral transcription [73]. Protease 3C has been shown to be critical for interaction with the cloverleaf structures found at the 5′ UTR of the viral genome to deliver the 3D to the replication complex [74]. They also indicated that since the function of 3C is required prior to 3D, a down-regulation in 3C would have a detrimental effect on viral transcription, as available 3D would not be able to carry out replication of CVB4 replication without the assistance of 3C. The authors' interpretation seems to be reasonable; however, according to the order (timing) of action for these enzymes, 2A cleaves the polyprotein prior to 3C cleavage. For this situation, it may be difficult to explain why the siRNAs targeting 2A did not achieve a more efficacious anti-CVB3 activity than siRNA targeting 3C. Obviously, many issues relating to the mechanisms of action need to be further studied. However, according to the present reports, one point is clear that 2A, 3C and 3D are three important targets for design anti-CVB3 siRNAs.

Viral structural protein VP1 was also a selected target for testing anti-CVB3 siRNAs; however, data from literature often showed less effectiveness of the siRNA targeting this structural gene compared to that targeting other genes [60, 65, 68]. Due to the absence of a proof-reading activity in 3D, the mutation rate for RNA viruses is as high as 10^{-3} -10^{-4} [75]. Thus, in recent years, the discovery of the occurrence of escape mutants due to siRNA treatment of HCV, poliovirus and HIV infections [76-78] greatly encouraged researchers to search for new approaches to counteract drug resistance. One direction is the application of multiple distinct siRNAs or a siRNA pool to target more than one target genes of the virus [79, 80]. The other direction is the identification of conserved cis-acting replication elements (CRE) [81]. Theoretically, the 5′ and 3′ UTRs are the ideal target regions for siRNAs as they harbor a number of conserved cis-acting elements. However, studies with poliovirus and CVB3 found that siRNA residing in these regions are less efficient than siRNAs targeting other regions (e.g., the coding region and particularly the non-structural coding region) in inducing antiviral activity [60, 77, 79, 82]. This low antiviral potency seems to be due to the highly ordered structure of the UTRs itself, as well as to the formation of the protein-RNA complexes in the region, which may block the access of the RISC complexes to its target sequences. To address this issue, Lee and coworkers selected a CRE within the coding region of 2C. Evaluation in HeLa cells demonstrated the down regulation of virus replication and attenuation of cytotoxicity in various strains and human isolates. Cells treated with this siRNA were resistant to the occurrence of viable escape mutants and showed sustained antiviral ability [83]. Based on this study, a similar experiment using siRNA targeting CRE of CVA24 2C was conducted and the authors reported similar observations [84]. These findings from *in vitro* studies were further strengthened by *in vivo* evaluation, in which recombinant lentivirus was employed to express shRNAs targeting the CRE of CVB3 2C. Mice injected intraperitoneally with recombinant lentiviruses had significant reductions in viral titers, viral myocarditis and proinflammatory cytokines as well as improved survival rate, after being challenged with CVB3 [85]. Recently, this CRE was further confirmed for a number of enteroviruses, by using a novel program and *in vitro* evaluation [86].

3.1.3.2. Targeting host cellular genes

Another approach to fight drug resistance caused by escape mutants is the selection of therapeutic targets within the host cellular genes that are involved in virus entry or viral replication. In this regard, the CAR receptor which is shared by CVB3 and adenovirus is an attractive candidate since both CVB3 and adenovirus are considered as the common causal agents of myocarditis. To date, two studies have been reported to silence CAR expression with specific siRNAs. One study reported that transfection of HeLa cells with siRNAs, siCAR2 or siCAR9, almost completely silenced the expression of CAR and that further analysis by viral plaque assay revealed ~60% reduction of CVB3 particle formation [67]. Another study, using cardiac-derived HL-1 cell line and primary neonatal cardiomyocytes (PNCMs) demonstrated that treatment with recombinant adenoviruses expressing shRNAs against CAR resulted in almost completely silencing of CAR expression in both HL-1 cells and PNCMs. CAR knockout resulted in inhibition of CVB3 infections by up to 97% in HL-1 and up to 90% in PNCMs. Adenoviruses were inhibited by only 75% in HL-1, but up to 92% in PNCMs [87].

Another host gene, the tissue inhibitor of matrix metalloproteinase-1 (TIMP-1), has been suggested to be a potential target for siRNA to ameliorate CVB3-induced myocarditis.

This suggestion is based on the investigation of Crocker and colleagues on a new role of TIMP-1 in exacerbating CVB-induced myocarditis. They found that TIMP-1 expression was induced in the myocardium by CVB3 infection. Surprisingly, TIMP-1 knockout mice exhibited a profound attenuation of myocarditis, with increased survival. The amelioration of disease in TIMP-1 knockout mice was not attributable to either an altered T-cell response to the virus nor to reduced viral replication. These data allowed the authors to propose and prove a novel function for TIMP-1. Its highly localized up-regulation might arrest the matrix metalloproteinase (MMP)-dependent migration of inflammatory cells at the sites of infection, thereby anatomically focusing the adaptive immune response. Finally, the benefits of TIMP-1 blockage in treating CVB3-induced myocarditis were confirmed by administration of siRNAs targeting TIMP-1, which diminished the disease. However, this improvement of the treatment is not due to changes of viral titers, as demonstrated by viral plaque assay [88].

Recently, active investigations on CVB3-induced signal transduction pathways have provided new avenues for the search of therapeutic targets for the treatment of myocarditis. Since CVB3, like other picornaviruses, requires the activation of certain signal pathways for initiating their life cycle, inactivation of some signal molecules in the signal cascade with specific siRNAs would block CVB3 replication. Such kind of studies that have been documented thus far include i) the knockdown of ubiquitin expression by siRNAs to down-regulate the ubiquitination and subsequent alteration of protein function and/or protein degradation [89]; ii) silencing of proteosome activator REG to inhibit the REG-mediated degradation of several important intracellular proteins [90], such as cyclin-dependent kinase inhibitors p21, p16 and tumor suppressor p53; and iii) knockdown of genes critical for autophagy formation including ATG7, Beeclin-1 and VPS34 [91]. Although these target genes mentioned above have been tested *in vitro* using specific siRNAs in signal transduction studies and showed promising outcomes, their potential serving as a therapeutic target for treatment of CVB3 infection needs further evaluation by pharmacological study in animal models.

3.1.4. Anti-CVB3 artificial miRNAs

miRNAs are a group of recently discovered new regulators of gene expression. These endogenous regulators control one third of human gene expression [92, 93]. Thus, endogenous miRNAs are important targets for gene therapy and artificial miRNAs (AmiRNA) are useful tools for inhibiting disease-causing gene expression [94, 95], which have been tested in numerous studies on the treatment of cancers, cardiovascular diseases, genetic diseases and other viral infections. To test its anti-CVB3 effect, we constructed three short hairpin AmiRNAs (AmiR-1, -2 and -3) targeting the stem-loop of the 3′ UTR of CVB3 with mismatches at the middle region of the target [96]. Transfection of HeLa cells showed over-expression of these mature AmiRNAs as determined by real time quantitative RT-PCR. After these AmiRNA-expressing cells were infected with CVB3, the viral

http://dx.doi.org/10.5772/54103

titers were reduced ~10 folds in cell cultures treated with AmiR-1 or AmiR-2 but not in those treated with AmiR-3, at 24 h post infection. Mutational analysis of the targeting sites of AmiRNAs demonstrated that the central region but not the seed region of AmiRNAs is more tolerant to target mutation. In this study we also performed targeted delivery of the AmiRNAs to host cells through ligand-receptor interactions. Recently, another group evaluated the antiviral activity of miR-342-5p in CVB3 infection of tissue culture cells. They found that miR-342-5p functions by targeting CVB3 2C region at nts 4989-5010, which is conserved in CVB type 1-5. Treatment of HeLa cells by transfection significantly inhibited viral RNA and protein synthesis. Mutation of the target site or using inhibitor of miR-342-5p decreased the antiviral effect *in vitro* [97].

In summary, the NA-based antivirals against CVB3 infection discussed above have shown great promise thus far (Table 1); however, none of them has reached the step for clinical trial. Many limitations such as drug stability, toxicity and targeted delivery need to be overcome before its addition to the list of clinical application.

4. Immunomodulatory therapy

As discussed above, the effectiveness of immunosuppressive therapy for viral myocarditis is controversial; we here focus the immunomodulatory therapy on immunoglobulin (Igs) treatment and immunoadsorption.

4.1. Immunoglobulin treatment

IgGs have already been shown to be efficacious treatments for Kawasaki disease [98], idiopathic thrombocytopenic purpura, and numerous neuroimmunologic disorders including Guillain-Barre syndrome [99]. The rationale to use IgG in viral infections results from their antiviral and immunomodulating effects. In the setting of viral myocarditis, IgGs can be utilized to suppress superfluous immune activation which may include an autoimmune component, but such treatment has shown conflicting results. IgGs prevented myocardial injury in experimental models of myocarditis [100, 101]. Even when administered in a delayed manner, IgG administration was able to limit scar formation and improve left ventricular (LV) function [101] or reduced pro-inflammatory TNF-α coupled with increased anti-inflammatory interleukins-1 and -10 [102]. More recently, Kishimoto et al [103] also showed improved heart function in adults with myocarditis and DCM. The same group recently showed that immunoglobulin treatment ameliorates myocardial injury in experimental autoimmune myocarditis associated with suppression of reactive oxygen species [104]. To date, however, there has only been one randomized clinical trial investigating IgG treatment in patients with myocarditis. McNamara et al [105] showed that, in a placebo-controlled prospective trial in patients with recent-onset DCM and myocarditis, intravenous immunoglobulin administration did not improve LV function.

Category	Target	Model system	Delivery route	Reference
PS-ASON	5' & 3'UTRs, IRES, start codon	HeLa cell, mice	Transfection	Wang 2001 (36)
PS-ASON	3'end of CVB3	HL-1 cells, mice	Transfection, IV injection	Yuan 2004 (37)
MOP-ASON	5' & 3'UTRs, IRES, start codon, minus strand	HeLa, HL-1 cell, mice	Transfection, IV injection	Yuan 2006 (38)
CpG oligomer	no	PBMCs	Treatment	Cong 2007 (39)
siRNA	2A, VP1, 3D	HeLa cells	Transfection	Yuan 2005 (60)
siRNA	2A	HeLa cells	pRNA vector	Zhang 2009 (62)
siRNA	2A	HeLa cells, mice	Hydrodynamic Transfection	Merl 2005 (63)
siRNA	2A	HeLa cells	Transfection	Racchi 2009 (64)
shRNA	3D	HeLa cells	Transfection of double expression plasmid	Schubert 2005 (66)
siRNA	3D, VP1	HeLa cells	Transfection	Ahn 2005 (65)
LNA-siRNA	3D	Cos-7 cells	Transfection	Schubert 2007 (61)
siRNA	siRNA pool	LLC-MK2 cells	Transfection	Nygardas 2009 (80)
shRNA	VP1, 3D, 5' & 3'UTR	Cos-7 cells, mice	Hydrodynamic Transfection	Kim J-Y 2008 (85)
siRNA & sCAR-Fc	3D	HMF	Transfection	Werk D 2009 (14)
shRNA	3D	HeLa, PNCMs, mice	Transduction, IV, AAV vector	Fechner 2008 (69)
siRNA (CVB4)	3D, 3C, 2A	RD cells	Transfection	Tan , 2010 (72)
shRNA	2C	Mice	IP injection, lentivirus vector	Lee 2007 (83)
shRNA (CVA24)	2C	HeLa, HCC	Transfection of plasmid	Jun 2008 (84)
siRNA (entero-viruses)	2C	HeLa, Vero cells	Transfection	Lee 2009 (86)
shRNA	CAR	HL-1, PNCMs	Adenovirus vector	Fechner 2007 (87)
siRNA	TIMP-1	Mice	IV injection	Crocker 2007 (88)
siRNA	CAR, 3D	HeLa,Cos-7 cells	Transfection	Werk 2005 (67)
siRNA	Ubiquitin	HeLa cells	Transfection	Si 2008 (89)
siRNA	ATG7, Beclin-, VPS34	HeLa cells	Transfection	Wong 2008 (91)
siRNA	Proteasome activator REGγ	HeLa cells	Transfection	Gao G 2010 (90)

Table 1. NA-based agents for the treatment of CVB3 infection

4.2. Immunoadsorption

The rationale for immunoadsorption is to lower concentration of cardiotoxic antibodies in patients plasma, and with serial treatments over 5 or more days, extract antibodies and immune complexes from the heart as well [106]. There is evidence that removal of circulating antibodies against cardiac proteins by immunoadsorption in DCM improved cardiac function [107] and reduced clinical and humoral markers of heart failure severity [108, 109] as well as improved hemodynamic parameters [110]. Further immunoadsorption decreased myocardial inflammation. In patients with inflammatory cardiomyopathy, LV systolic function improved after protein A immunoadsorption [111]. Recently, Nagatomo et al reported that immunoadsorption using IgG3-specific tryptophan column for patients with refractory heart failure due to DCM is a safe treatment and has shown short term efficacy. Long term follow-up is needed to confirm the effects on cardiac function and on morbidity/mortality in such patients [112]. Another recent study demonstrated that immunoadsorption treatment improved endothelial function in patients with chronic inflammatory DCM. This effect is associated with a significant drop in circulating microparticles [113].

5. Antiviral treatment

5.1. Compounds inhibiting viral replication

As mentioned earlier, ribavirin is a frequently used antiviral agent. This agent is a nucleoside analogue and can block viral transcription elongation and thus can be used to inhibit a number of RNA viral infections, including CVB3 [114, 115]. Recently, new antiviral compounds have been synthesized. Harki et al. synthesized some cytidine analogues and one of them, 5-nitrocytidine, decreased CVB3 titer in infected cells, with 12-fold higher efficiency than ribavirin, but so far the *in vivo* evaluation has not been reported [116]. Other strategies for antiviral compound design are inhibitors of viral protease, RNA-dependent RNA polymerase or other nonstructural proteins, such as guanidine hypochloride, HBB, MRL-1237 and TBZE-02, which interact with viral 2C protein resulting in inhibition of viral RNA transcription.

Nitrooxide (NO) donor is another form of antiviral agents interfering with viral nonstructural proteins. They inhibit enterovirus proteases 2A and 3C [109, 117]. The NO donors nitroglycerin (GTN) and isosorbide dinitrate (ISDN) can suppress CVB3 replication by inhibiting viral proteases *in vitro*. Further, *in vivo* study showed that GTN significantly reduced myocarditis after administration by decreasing immune cell infiltration and tissue fibrosis up to 14 day post infection [111]. In another study using a CVB3 myocarditis mouse model, treatment with NO-metoprolol showed enhanced therapeutic benefit compared to metoprolol, with significant reduction of viral RNA synthesis, body weight loss, infiltration and fibrosis score [118]. Interestingly, another study using cinnamaldehyde, which can reduce plasma nitric oxide (NO) content, also showed the effectiveness in treatment of CVB3 myocarditis. This compound also reduced NF-κB, inducible nitric oxide synthase and TLR4 expression. Thus, the underlying mechanism is likely by inhibiting the TLR4-NF-κB signal transduction pathway [119]. Recently, a protein-based CVB3 protease 3C inhibitor, 3CPI, demonstrated that treatment by way of a micro-osmotic pump delivery significantly inhibited viral proliferation, and attenuated myocardial inflammations, subsequent fibrosis, and CVB3-induced mortality *in vivo* [120].

5.2. Interferons (IFNs)

IFNs are critical cytokines of the innate immune response released in response to stimuli with particular importance in viral infection. IFN signal through one of two receptor groups which dictates their subtype IFN-alpha and IFN-beta are of type I and IFN-gamma is of type II. Type I IFNs trigger critical antiviral responses whereas, type II IFNs contribute to immune enhancement and modulation including an important role in macrophage activation. The best studied of these proteins is the IFN-gamma. Infections in IFN-gamma-deficient mice showed that IFN-gamma triggers release of IL-1, IL-4 and transforming growth factor, the latter being sentinel to development of cardiac fibrosis [121]. Notably, expression of IFN-gamma by IFN-gamma recombinant CVB3 vector protected mice against infection of lethal CVB3H3 variant by decreasing the viral load and spread as well as tissue destruction when given prior to or directly after viral infection [122, 123].

Type I IFNs have also shown promise in the treatment of viral myocarditis. IFN-alpha is known to trigger a number of biological cascades to inhibit virus infection. IFN-alpha was used successfully to treat two patients with acute enterovirus-induced myocarditis [123]. As well, IFN-beta therapy has been used to improve the prognosis for patients with DCM [124]. Recently, experimental evidence has suggested that IFN-beta can also be used as an antiviral treatment and can improve outcome in viral myocarditis [125, 126]. These studies showed that treatment with IFN-beta resulted in an elimination of cardiac viral load, protected cardiomyocytes against injury and decreased inflammatory cell infiltrates. In a placebo controlled, randomized, double-blind, phase II trial (BICC-study), 143 patients with inflammatory DCM and viral myocarditis were treated with IFN-beta-1b and showed significant reduction of viral load (enterovirus) in myocardium; however, complete viral elimination (parvovirus B19) was not achieved in all patients [127]. This is probably due to that this virus responds less well upon IFN-beta treatment. Novel IFN amplification using poly(inosinic acid)-poly(cytidylic acid) [poly(IC)], IFN-alpha-2b, pegylated IFN-alpha-2b (PEG-INTRON-alpha-2b), and ampligen have proved successful in blocking virus infection [128]. Oral administration of IFN-alpha-2b expressing bacteria (*B. longum*) also protects mice against CVB3-induced myocarditis [129]. In addition, type I interferons induced by modified 3p-siRNA specifically targeting CVB3 genome significantly reduced viral load and damage of the heart [130].

5.3. Soluble receptor analogues

Another similar strategy in developing antiviral agents is to block viral entry by utilization of recombinant soluble protein of CAR receptor. Detailed review can be found in a recent article [21]. Soluble receptor analogues bind to the virus before the viral binding to its receptor, thus preventing binding of virus and subsequent entry to the target cells. Several research groups designed and produced this type of analogues by recombinant DNA technology to increase its efficiency. The most common strategy is the modification of the protein by fusion of virus binding domain on the receptor, CAR or DAF, with the C-terminus of the human IgG1 Fc region, resulting in a dimeric antibody-like molecule. This modification greatly enhanced the solubility and stability of the fusion protein [13, 15, 131-133]; as well as increased the efficiency in viral neutralization [134]. However, one study reported the possible side effects caused by this approach, which demonstrated that after treatment with recombinant CAR4/7, animal showed aggravated myocardium inflammation, tissue damage and presence of CAR-specific antibody. The possible mechanism leading to this problem may be due to the bacteria-produced recombinant protein altered the glycosylation pattern and increased the immunogenicity [135]. Recently, another study simultaneously applied soluble CAR-Fc and siRNA targeting CVB3 genome exerted synergistic antiviral activity in the treatment of a persistently infected cardiac cell line *in vitro* [14].

6. Natural products

Natural products occupy tremendous chemical structural space – unmatched by any other small molecule families – possess a range of biological activities, remain the best sources of drugs and drug leads, and serve as outstanding small molecule probes for dissecting fundamental biological processes [136, 137]. Natural products are evolutionarily optimized to be drug-like. They are generally more potent and specific than synthetic molecules, suggesting increased binding affinities for their cognate protein receptors. This characteristic may be attributed to the fact that natural products are biosynthetically made through repeated interaction with modulating enzymes; thus their ability to interact with biological macromolecules is intrinsic to their structures. In addition, they may result from a complex evolutionary interaction between co-occupants of an ecological niche, resulting in the optimization of natural products in a process that is inaccessible to synthetic compounds [138-140].

The natural products, such as *Astragalus membranaceus, Salviae miltiorrhizae, Sophorae flavescentis* and *Phyllanthus emblica* or Chinese proprietary medicines, such as Shenmai, Shuanghuangkian and Qishaowuwei, have been long known to be effective in treating viral myocarditis. However, the components of the medicine and the mode of action are largely unknown [141]. Recent years, emerging studies focused on the isolation of the major component of the medicine and the mechanisms of action. Astragaloside IV is probably the most studied natural compound in anti-myocarditis caused by viral infection. Two groups isolated this compound from *Astragalus membranaceus* and *Radix Astragali* respectively and all showed the effectiveness of this component in treatment of CVB3 infection of the heart. One group demonstrated that treatment could significantly decrease virus load, mononuclear cell infiltration and cardiomyocyte injury in mice. They further found that astragaloside IV exerted antiviral effects against CVB3 by upregulating IFN-gamma expression [142]. The other group showed that astragalus treatment significantly decreased the fibrosis of the heart tissue and increased the mouse survival rate; further analysis revealed that this cardioprotective effect is largely due to the inhibition of the TGF-beta 1-Smad signaling in DCM [143]. Sophoridine, an alkaloid extracted from *Sophora flavescens*, has been evaluated in mice and rats. The results showed that sophoridine treatment obviously decreased viral titer and enhanced mRNA expression of IL-1 and IFN-gamma but decreased TNF-alpha. They concluded that sophoridine itself but not its metabolites is responsible for its antiviral activity by regulating cytokine expression [144]. Recently, another natural product phyllaemblicin B, the main sesquiterpenoid glyside isolated from roots of *Phyllanthus emblica*, was reported to reduce CVB3-iduced apoptosis both *in vitro* and *in vivo*. In CVB3 myocarditis mouse model, this compound reduced CVB3 titer, decreased activities of LDH and CK in murine serum, and alleviated pathological damage of the myocardium [145].

7. Cellular cardiomyoplasty

The critical loss of functional cardiomyocytes causes a severe deterioration of contractility, which eventually results in heart failure. To reverse the myocardial injuries in disease progression, the damaged, hypocontractile and necrotic myocytes need be replaced. Although in contrast to the long-standing dogma that mammalian heart loses capability of proliferation in injuries after birth, there is much evidence now to support a degree of regeneration in postnatal human heart. Regardless of whether the proliferating myocytes are derived from the resident cardiomyocytes or circulating stem cells, it is obvious that this self-renew mechanism is not sufficient in amount to prevent or block the heart failure.

Cellular cardiomyoplasty (CCM) is now emerging as one of the most promising therapeutic techniques for the augmentation and regeneration of injured myocardium [146]. The strategy is to introduce less differentiated or undifferentiated cells, or *in vitro* derived cardiomyocytes into injured heart to mediate repair of chronically injured myocardium [147]. Cells of various origins and stages of differentiation, but with the capability of differentiating into a contractile phenotype have been utilized. The most frequently referred cell types for such treatment are skeletal myoblast, embryonic stem cells, and bone marrow cells which contain lineages of hematopoietic and mesenchymal stem cells [148].

All transplanted cell lines mentioned above showed some improvements on myocardial regional and/or global function in a variety of animal models and some have been investigated in clinical trials. Although the mechanism of improved cardiac function with implanted cells requires further study, the following evidence may help us to understand the general therapeutic process: i) systolic contraction generated by implanted cardiomyocytes; ii) alteration and attenuation of deleterious ventricular remodeling; iii) induction of angiogenesis by released growth factors such as vascular endothelial growth factor, basic fibroblast growth factor, and angiopoietin-1.

To date, a number of studies have been conducted for the treatment of myocardial infarction or chromic myocardial ischemia, only a few experimental cell-based studies are directed at treating nonischemic cardiomyopathy [149, 150]. The treatment studies for virus-induced viral myocarditis or DCM is even fewer. Here we only found two reports on the CVB3-induced myocarditis. The pioneer work by van Linthout and co-workers demonstrated that mesenchymal stem cells (MSCs) are potential therapeutic cells for the CVB3-viral myocarditis [151]. This finding is largely based on that these cells express a low level of CAR receptor and thus are not sensitive to CVB3 infection. In co-culture experiments with the cardiomyocytes HL-1, MSCs reduced CVB3-induced cell apoptosis and oxidative stress. Furthermore, MSCs diminished viral progeny release by approximately 5-fold. Importantly, intravenous injection of MSCs decreased cardiac apoptosis and improved LV function in a murine CVB3 myocarditis model. A detailed study on the mechanism revealed that the protective effect of MSCs is mediated in an NO-dependent manner and requires priming via IFN-gamma. Another recent study using cardiac-derived adherent proliferating cells (CAPs) showed similar results as that using MSCs [152]. CAPs only minimally express both CAR and DAF receptors, which translates to minimal CVB3 copy numbers, and without viral particle release after infection. Co-culture of CAPs with CVB3-infected HL-1 cells resulted in a reduction of CVB3-induced HL-1 cell apoptosis and viral progeny release. In addition, CAPs have immunomodulatory feature and can lead to a decrease in CVB3 load, myocyte death and an improvement in LV contractility parameters in murine acute CVB3 myocarditis. CAPs exert protective effects in an NO-and IL-10-dependnet manner and require IFN-gamma for their activation.

Despite many questions regarding stem cell plasticity have not been answered, exploratory clinical trials are currently underway with both skeletal myoblasts [153, 154] and bone marrow-derived cells [155, 156]. It is estimated that more than 15 patients have been treated with CCM worldwide, and the number of patients treated with autologous skeletal myoblasts is equivalent to those treated with bone marrow cells [156]. These preliminary results of CCM are encouraging. However, the potential for this treatment will heavily depend on conducting more rigorously controlled and randomized clinical trials with appropriate endpoints to show a clear therapeutic benefit of this approach. In addition, for CCM to become a widely accepted therapy in the future, fundamental questions such as best cell source, appropriate cell dose, timing of implantation, optimum delivery mode, mechanism of action, electrical and mechanical integration, cell survival and long term fate of transplanted cells, need to be addressed.

8. Concluding remarks

Since the last decades, a number of new strategies have been emerged in drug development for treatment of viral myocarditis and its sequela DCM, which are summarized in Figure 2. As myocarditis can be induced by a number of viruses, rapid and timely pathogen identification is critically important for guiding early and targeted treatments. Certainly, rapid, sensitive and specific detection of a particular virus or even viral subtype in human samples by detection of virus-specific genes would facilitate targeted treatments. This is particularly crucial for the treatments using nucleic acid-based antiviral agents targeting viral RNA.

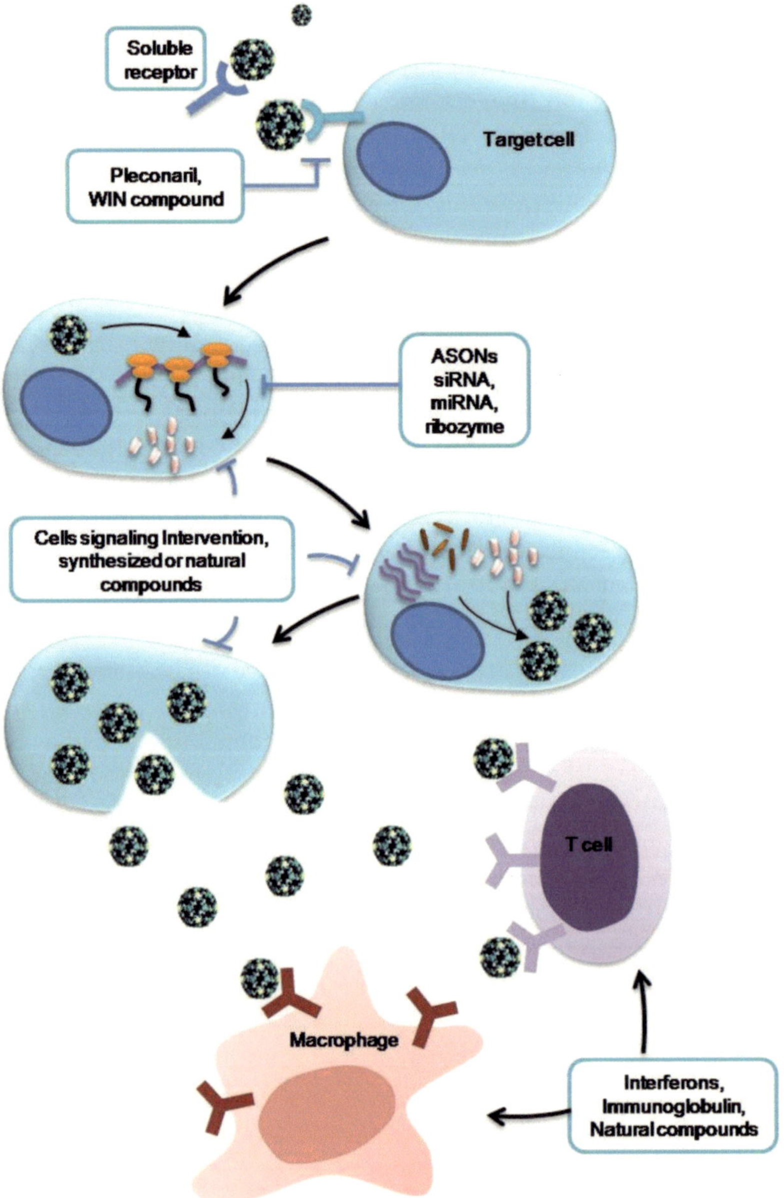

Figure 2. Antiviral strategies for CVB3 infection. The potential therapeutic targets in viral life cycle and the subsequent inflammatory response are indicated for different antiviral agents.

As CVB3 is a RNA virus and has a high mutation rate, drug resistant mutations pose potential obstacles. Therefore, drug targeting on viral proteins for viral replication is another choice for drug design. For example, the inhibition of RNA-dependent RNA polymerase or proteases of CVB3 may offer great promise since their functions are essential for the virus but not for the cell. In the treatment of infection using nucleic acid-based antiviral agents,

http://dx.doi.org/10.5772/54103

simultaneous application of several drugs may achieve synergistic effects and also reduce the emergence of drug resistance. In addition, combination with the non-nucleic acid-based drugs, such as interferon or soluble receptor, may also achieve the same goal. Recent emerging of the artificial microRNA technology provides another strategy for overcoming drug resistance because miRNA targeting requires partial complementation and is more tolerant to target mutation than siRNA. In searching for new antiviral drugs, although the natural products have long been known to be valuable sources of such agents, progresses in this area of research are not significant as compared to other areas of drug development. Thus more efforts should be made in the screen of the natural antiviral compounds. For end-stage therapy, in light of the preliminary clinical studies, CCM is no doubt an exciting area. We look forward with great anticipation to future clinical studies and a greater understanding of the mechanism of action, which will potentially lead to clinical applications.

Acknowledgements

The work was supported by a China-Canada (CIHR) Joint Health Research Initiative grant. Xin Ye is supported by a University Graduate Fellowship.

Author details

Decheng Yang[1,2], Huifang Mary Zhang[1,2], Xin Ye[1,2], Lixin Zhang[3] and Huanqin Dai[3]

1 Department of Pathology and Laboratory Medicine, University of British Columbia, Canada

2 The Institute for Heart + Lung Health at St. Paul's Hospital, Vancouver, Canada

3 Chinese Academy of Sciences Key Laboratory of Pathogenic Microbiology and Immunology, Institute of Microbiology, Beijing, PRC

References

[1] Andreoletti, L., et al. Viral causes of human myocarditis. Archive of Cardiovascular Diseases, 2009; 102(6-7) 559-68.

[2] Horwitz, M.S., et al. Transforming growth factor-beta inhibits coxsackievirus-mediated autoimmune myocarditis. Viral Immunology, 2006; 19(4) 722-33.

[3] Blauwet, L.A. and Cooper, L.T. Myocarditis. Progress in Cardiovascular Diseases, 2010; 52(4) 274-88.

[4] Hosenpud, J.D., et al. The Registry of the International Society for Heart and Lung Transplantation: eighteenth Official Report-2001. Journal of Heart and Lung Transplantation, 2001; 20(8) 805-15.

[5] Drory, Y., et al. Sudden unexpected death in persons less than 40 years of age. American Journal of Cardiology, 1991; 68(13) 1388-92.

[6] Verma, B., Bhattacharyya, S., and Das, S. Polypyrimidine tract-binding protein interacts with coxsackievirus B3 RNA and influences its translation. Journal of General Virology; 91(Pt 5) 1245-55.

[7] Cheung, P., et al. Specific interaction of HeLa cell proteins with coxsackievirus B3 3'UTR: La autoantigen binds the 3' and 5'UTR independently of the poly(A) tail. Cellular Microbiology, 2007; 9(7) 1705-15.

[8] Liu, Z., et al. Structural and functional analysis of the 5' untranslated region of coxsackievirus B3 RNA: In vivo translational and infectivity studies of full-length mutants. Virology, 1999; 265(2) 206-17.

[9] Yang, D., et al. In vitro mutational and inhibitory analysis of the cis-acting translational elements within the 5' untranslated region of coxsackievirus B3: potential targets for antiviral action of antisense oligomers. Virology, 1997; 228(1) 63-73.

[10] Melchers, W.J., et al. Kissing of the two predominant hairpin loops in the coxsackie B virus 3' untranslated region is the essential structural feature of the origin of replication required for negative-strand RNA synthesis. Journal of Virology, 1997; 71(1) 686-96.

[11] Wang, J., et al. Structural requirements of the higher order RNA kissing element in the enteroviral 3'UTR. Nucleic Acids Research, 1999; 27(2) 485-90.

[12] Raschperger, E., et al. The coxsackie- and adenovirus receptor (CAR) is an in vivo marker for epithelial tight junctions, with a potential role in regulating permeability and tissue homeostasis. Experimental Cell Research, 2006; 312(9) 1566-80.

[13] Pinkert, S., et al. Prevention of cardiac dysfunction in acute coxsackievirus B3 cardiomyopathy by inducible expression of a soluble coxsackievirus-adenovirus receptor. Circulation, 2009; 120(23) 2358-66.

[14] Werk, D., et al. Combination of soluble coxsackievirus-adenovirus receptor and anti-coxsackievirus siRNAs exerts synergistic antiviral activity against coxsackievirus B3. Antiviral Research, 2009; 83(3) 298-306.

[15] Yanagawa, B., et al. Soluble recombinant coxsackievirus and adenovirus receptor abrogates coxsackievirus b3-mediated pancreatitis and myocarditis in mice. Journal of Infectious Diseases, 2004; 189(8) 1431-9.

[16] Freimuth, P., Philipson, L., and Carson, S.D. The coxsackievirus and adenovirus receptor. Current Topics in Microbiology and Immunology, 2008; 323 67-87.

[17] Shafren, D.R., Williams, D.T., and Barry, R.D. A decay-accelerating factor-binding strain of coxsackievirus B3 requires the coxsackievirus-adenovirus receptor protein to mediate lytic infection of rhabdomyosarcoma cells. Journal of Virology, 1997; 71(12) 9844-8.

[18] Schultz, J.C., et al. Diagnosis and treatment of viral myocarditis. Mayo Clinic Proceedings, 2009; 84(11) 1001-9.

[19] Dennert, R., Crijns, H.J., and Heymans, S. Acute viral myocarditis. European Heart Journal, 2008; 29(17) 2073-82.

[20] Rose, N.R. Myocarditis: infection versus autoimmunity. Journal of Clinical Immunology, 2009; 29(6) 730-7.

[21] Fechner, H., et al. Pharmacological and biological antiviral therapeutics for cardiac coxsackievirus infections. Molecules, 2011; 16(10) 8475-503.

[22] Kindermann, I., et al. Update on myocarditis. Journal of the American College of Cardiology, 2012; 59(9) 779-92.

[23] Cooper, L.T., et al. The role of endomyocardial biopsy in the management of cardiovascular disease: a scientific statement from the American Heart Association, the American College of Cardiology, and the European Society of Cardiology. Endorsed by the Heart Failure Society of America and the Heart Failure Association of the European Society of Cardiology. Journal of the American College of Cardiology, 2007; 50(19) 1914-31.

[24] Frustaci, A., et al. Immunosuppressive therapy for active lymphocytic myocarditis: virological and immunologic profile of responders versus nonresponders. Circulation, 2003; 107(6) 857-63.

[25] Groarke, J.M. and Pevear, D.C. Attenuated virulence of pleconaril-resistant coxsackievirus B3 variants. Journal of Infectious Diseases, 1999; 179(6) 1538-41.

[26] Kaiser, L., Crump, C.E., and Hayden, F.G. In vitro activity of pleconaril and AG7088 against selected serotypes and clinical isolates of human rhinoviruses. Antiviral Research, 2000; 47(3) 215-20.

[27] Reisdorph, N., et al. Human rhinovirus capsid dynamics is controlled by canyon flexibility. Virology, 2003; 314(1) 34-44.

[28] Fohlman, J., et al. Antiviral treatment with WIN 54 954 reduces mortality in murine coxsackievirus B3 myocarditis. Circulation, 1996; 94(9) 2254-9.

[29] Fox, M.P., Otto, M.J., and McKinlay, M.A. Prevention of rhinovirus and poliovirus uncoating by WIN 51711, a new antiviral drug. Antimicrobial Agents and Chemotherapy, 1986; 30(1) 110-6.

[30] Lewis, J.K., et al. Antiviral agent blocks breathing of the common cold virus. Proceedings of the National Academy of Sciences of the United States of America, 1998; 95(12) 6774-8.

[31] Pevear, D.C., et al. Activity of pleconaril against enteroviruses. Antimicrobial Agents and Chemotherapy, 1999; 43(9) 2109-15.

[32] Schmidtke, M., et al. New pleconaril and [(biphenyloxy)propyl]isoxazole derivatives with substitutions in the central ring exhibit antiviral activity against pleconaril-resistant coxsackievirus B3. Antiviral Research, 2009; 81(1) 56-63.

[33] Stein, D., et al. A specificity comparison of four antisense types: morpholino, 2'-O-methyl RNA, DNA, and phosphorothioate DNA. Antisense and Nucleic Acid Drug Development, 1997; 7(3) 151-7.

[34] Hoke, G.D., et al. Effects of phosphorothioate capping on antisense oligonucleotide stability, hybridization and antiviral efficacy versus herpes simplex virus infection. Nucleic Acids Research, 1991; 19(20) 5743-8.

[35] Cotten, M., et al. 2'-O-methyl, 2'-O-ethyl oligoribonucleotides and phosphorothioate oligodeoxyribonucleotides as inhibitors of the in vitro U7 snRNP-dependent mRNA processing event. Nucleic Acids Research, 1991; 19(10) 2629-35.

[36] Wang, A., et al. Specific inhibition of coxsackievirus B3 translation and replication by phosphorothioate antisense oligodeoxynucleotides. Antimicrobial Agents and Chemotherapy, 2001; 45(4) 1043-52.

[37] Yuan, J., et al. A phosphorothioate antisense oligodeoxynucleotide specifically inhibits coxsackievirus B3 replication in cardiomyocytes and mouse hearts. Laboratory Investigation, 2004; 84(6) 703-14.

[38] Yuan, J., et al. Inhibition of coxsackievirus B3 in cell cultures and in mice by peptide-conjugated morpholino oligomers targeting the internal ribosome entry site. Journal of Virology, 2006; 80(23) 11510-9.

[39] Cong, Z., et al. A CpG oligodeoxynucleotide inducing anti-coxsackie B3 virus activity in human peripheral blood mononuclear cells. FEMS Immunology and Medical Microbiology, 2007; 51(1) 26-34.

[40] Peracchi, A. Prospects for antiviral ribozymes and deoxyribozymes. Reviews in Medical Virology, 2004; 14(1) 47-64.

[41] Matsumori, A. Hepatitis C virus infection and cardiomyopathies. Circulation Research, 2005; 96(2) 144-7.

[42] Matsumori, A., et al. Myocarditis and heart failure associated with hepatitis C virus infection. Journal of Cardiac Failure, 2006; 12(4) 293-8.

[43] Macejak, D.G., et al. Inhibition of hepatitis C virus (HCV)-RNA-dependent translation and replication of a chimeric HCV poliovirus using synthetic stabilized ribozymes. Hepatology, 2000; 31(3) 769-76.

[44] Macejak, D.G., et al. Enhanced antiviral effect in cell culture of type 1 interferon and ribozymes targeting HCV RNA. Journal of Viral Hepatitis, 2001; 8(6) 400-5.

[45] Gonzalez-Carmona, M.A., et al. Hammerhead ribozymes with cleavage site specificity for NUH and NCH display significant anti-hepatitis C viral effect in vitro and in recombinant HepG2 and CCL13 cells. Journal of Hepatology, 2006; 44(6) 1017-25.

[46] Bennasser, Y., et al. Evidence that HIV-1 encodes an siRNA and a suppressor of RNA silencing. Immunity, 2005; 22(5) 607-19.

[47] Berkhout, B. and Jeang, K.T. RISCy business: MicroRNAs, pathogenesis, and viruses. Journal of Biological Chemistry, 2007; 282(37) 26641-5.

[48] Cullen, B.R. Is RNA interference involved in intrinsic antiviral immunity in mammals? Nature Immunology, 2006; 7(6) 563-7.

[49] Lecellier, C.H., et al. A cellular microRNA mediates antiviral defense in human cells. Science, 2005; 308(5721) 557-60.

[50] Otsuka, M., et al. Hypersusceptibility to vesicular stomatitis virus infection in Dicer1-deficient mice is due to impaired miR24 and miR93 expression. Immunity, 2007; 27(1) 123-34.

[51] Hannon, G.J. RNA interference. Nature, 2002; 418(6894) 244-51.

[52] Tomari, Y. and Zamore, P.D. Perspective: machines for RNAi. Genes and Development, 2005; 19(5) 517-29.

[53] Caudy, A.A., et al. A micrococcal nuclease homologue in RNAi effector complexes. Nature, 2003; 425(6956) 411-4.

[54] Brennecke, J., et al. Principles of microRNA-target recognition. PLoS Biology, 2005; 3(3) e85.

[55] Grimson, A., et al. MicroRNA targeting specificity in mammals: determinants beyond seed pairing. Molecular Cell, 2007; 27(1) 91-105.

[56] Krek, A., et al. Combinatorial microRNA target predictions. Nature Genetics, 2005; 37(5) 495-500.

[57] Lewis, B.P., et al. Prediction of mammalian microRNA targets. Cell, 2003; 115(7) 787-98.

[58] Doench, J.G., Petersen, C.P., and Sharp, P.A. siRNAs can function as miRNAs. Genes and Development, 2003; 17(4) 438-42.

[59] Parker, J.S., Roe, S.M., and Barford, D. Structural insights into mRNA recognition from a PIWI domain-siRNA guide complex. Nature, 2005; 434(7033) 663-6.

[60] Yuan, J., et al. Inhibition of coxsackievirus B3 replication by small interfering RNAs requires perfect sequence match in the central region of the viral positive strand. Journal of Virology, 2005; 79(4) 2151-9.

[61] Schubert, S., et al. Strand-specific silencing of a picornavirus by RNA interference: evidence for the superiority of plus-strand specific siRNAs. Antiviral Research, 2007; 73(3) 197-205.

[62] Zhang, H.M., et al. Targeted delivery of anti-coxsackievirus siRNAs using ligand-conjugated packaging RNAs. Antiviral Research, 2009; 83(3) 307-16.

[63] Merl, S., et al. Targeting 2A protease by RNA interference attenuates coxsackieviral cytopathogenicity and promotes survival in highly susceptible mice. Circulation, 2005; 111(13) 1583-92.

[64] Racchi, G., et al. Targeting of protease 2A genome by single and multiple siRNAs as a strategy to impair CVB3 life cycle in permissive HeLa cells. Methods and Findings in Experimental and Clinical Pharmacology, 2009; 31(2) 63-70.

[65] Ahn, J., et al. A small interfering RNA targeting coxsackievirus B3 protects permissive HeLa cells from viral challenge. Journal of Virology, 2005; 79(13) 8620-4.

[66] Schubert, S., et al. Maintaining inhibition: siRNA double expression vectors against coxsackieviral RNAs. Journal of Molecular Biology, 2005; 346(2) 457-65.

[67] Werk, D., et al. Developing an effective RNA interference strategy against a plus-strand RNA virus: silencing of coxsackievirus B3 and its cognate coxsackievirus-adenovirus receptor. Biological Chemistry, 2005; 386(9) 857-63.

[68] Kim, J.Y., et al. Expression of short hairpin RNAs against the coxsackievirus B3 exerts potential antiviral effects in Cos-7 cells and in mice. Virus Research, 2007; 125(1) 9-13.

[69] Fechner, H., et al. Cardiac-targeted RNA interference mediated by an AAV9 vector improves cardiac function in coxsackievirus B3 cardiomyopathy. Journal of Molecular Medicine, 2008; 86(9) 987-97.

[70] Chau, D.H., et al. Coxsackievirus B3 proteases 2A and 3C induce apoptotic cell death through mitochondrial injury and cleavage of eIF4GI but not DAP5/p97/NAT1. Apoptosis, 2007; 12(3) 513-24.

[71] Leong, L.E., Cornell, C.T., and Semler, B.L. Processing determinants and functions of cleavage products of picornavirus polyproteins. in: Semler, B.L. and Wimmer, E. (ed.) Molecular biology of picornaviruses. Washington, D.C.: ASM Press; 2002. p187-197.

[72] Tan, E.L., Wong, A.P., and Poh, C.L. Development of potential antiviral strategy against coxsackievirus B4. Virus Research, 2010; 150(1-2) 85-92.

[73] Parsley, T.B., Cornell, C.T., and Semler, B.L. Modulation of the RNA binding and protein processing activities of poliovirus polypeptide 3CD by the viral RNA polymerase domain. Journal of Biological Chemistry, 1999; 274(18) 12867-76.

[74] Leong, L.E., Walker, P.A., and Porter, A.G. Human rhinovirus-14 protease 3C (3Cpro) binds specifically to the 5'-noncoding region of the viral RNA. Evidence that

3Cpro has different domains for the RNA binding and proteolytic activities. Journal of Biological Chemistry, 1993; 268(34) 25735-9.

[75] Cann, A.J., editor. Principles of Molecular Virology. Waltham: Academic Press; 2005.

[76] Boden, D., et al. Human immunodeficiency virus type 1 escape from RNA interference. Journal of Virology, 2003; 77(21) 11531-5.

[77] Gitlin, L., Stone, J.K., and Andino, R. Poliovirus escape from RNA interference: short interfering RNA-target recognition and implications for therapeutic approaches. Journal of Virology, 2005; 79(2) 1027-35.

[78] Wilson, J.A. and Richardson, C.D. Hepatitis C virus replicons escape RNA interference induced by a short interfering RNA directed against the NS5b coding region. Journal of Virology, 2005; 79(11) 7050-8.

[79] Merl, S. and Wessely, R. Anti-coxsackieviral efficacy of RNA interference is highly dependent on genomic target selection and emergence of escape mutants. Oligonucleotides, 2007; 17(1) 44-53.

[80] Nygardas, M., et al. Inhibition of coxsackievirus B3 and related enteroviruses by antiviral short interfering RNA pools produced using phi6 RNA-dependent RNA polymerase. Journal of General Virology, 2009; 90(Pt 10) 2468-73.

[81] van Ooij, M.J., et al. Structural and functional characterization of the coxsackievirus B3 CRE(2C): role of CRE(2C) in negative- and positive-strand RNA synthesis. Journal of General Virology, 2006; 87(Pt 1) 103-13.

[82] Saleh, M.C., Van Rij, R.P., and Andino, R. RNA silencing in viral infections: insights from poliovirus. Virus Research, 2004; 102(1) 11-7.

[83] Lee, H.S., et al. Universal and mutation-resistant anti-enteroviral activity: potency of small interfering RNA complementary to the conserved cis-acting replication element within the enterovirus coding region. Journal of General Virology, 2007; 88(Pt 7) 2003-12.

[84] Jun, E.J., et al. Antiviral potency of a siRNA targeting a conserved region of coxsackievirus A24. Biochemical and Biophysical Research Communications, 2008; 376(2) 389-94.

[85] Kim, Y.J., et al. Recombinant lentivirus-delivered short hairpin RNAs targeted to conserved coxsackievirus sequences protect against viral myocarditis and improve survival rate in an animal model. Virus Genes, 2008; 36(1) 141-6.

[86] Lee, H.S., et al. A novel program to design siRNAs simultaneously effective to highly variable virus genomes. Biochemical and Biophysical Research Communications, 2009; 384(4) 431-5.

[87] Fechner, H., et al. Coxsackievirus B3 and adenovirus infections of cardiac cells are efficiently inhibited by vector-mediated RNA interference targeting their common receptor. Gene Therapy, 2007; 14(12) 960-71.

[88] Crocker, S.J., et al. Amelioration of coxsackievirus B3-mediated myocarditis by inhibition of tissue inhibitors of matrix metalloproteinase-1. American Journal of Pathology, 2007; 171(6) 1762-73.

[89] Si, X., et al. Ubiquitination is required for effective replication of coxsackievirus B3. PLoS ONE, 2008; 3(7) e2585.

[90] Gao, G., et al. Proteasome activator REGgamma enhances coxsackieviral infection by facilitating p53 degradation. Journal of Virology, 2010; 84(21) 11056-66.

[91] Wong, J., et al. Autophagosome supports coxsackievirus B3 replication in host cells. Journal of Virology, 2008; 82(18) 9143-53.

[92] Bartel, D.P. MicroRNAs: target recognition and regulatory functions. Cell, 2009; 136(2) 215-33.

[93] Liu, Q. and Paroo, Z. Biochemical principles of small RNA pathways. Annual Review of Biochemistry, 2010; 79 295-319.

[94] Liu, Z., Sall, A., and Yang, D. MicroRNA: An emerging therapeutic target and intervention tool. International Journal of Molecular Sciences, 2008; 9(6) 978-99.

[95] Sall, A., et al. MicroRNAs-based therapeutic strategy for virally induced diseases. Current Drug Discovery Technologies, 2008; 5(1) 49-58.

[96] Ye, X., et al. Targeted delivery of mutant tolerant anti-coxsackievirus artificial microRNAs using folate conjugated bacteriophage Phi29 pRNA. PLoS ONE, 2011; 6(6) e21215.

[97] Wang, L., et al. MiR-342-5p suppresses coxsackievirus B3 biosynthesis by targeting the 2C-coding region. Antiviral Research, 2012; 93(2) 270-9.

[98] Furusho, K., et al. High-dose intravenous gammaglobulin for Kawasaki disease. Lancet, 1984; 2(8411) 1055-8.

[99] Latov, N., et al. Use of intravenous gamma globulins in neuroimmunologic diseases. Journal of Allergy and Clinical Immunology, 2001; 108(4 Suppl) S126-32.

[100] Weller, A.H., Hall, M., and Huber, S.A. Polyclonal immunoglobulin therapy protects against cardiac damage in experimental coxsackievirus-induced myocarditis. European Heart Journal, 1992; 13(1) 115-9.

[101] Takada, H., Kishimoto, C., and Hiraoka, Y. Therapy with immunoglobulin suppresses myocarditis in a murine coxsackievirus B3 model. Antiviral and anti-inflammatory effects. Circulation, 1995; 92(6) 1604-11.

[102] Gullestad, L., et al. Immunomodulating therapy with intravenous immunoglobulin in patients with chronic heart failure. Circulation, 2001; 103(2) 220-5.

[103] Kishimoto, C., et al. Treatment of acute inflammatory cardiomyopathy with intravenous immunoglobulin ameliorates left ventricular function associated with suppres-

sion of inflammatory cytokines and decreased oxidative stress. International Journal of Cardiology, 2003; 91(2-3) 173-8.

[104] Fan, F., et al. Effect of PGE2 on DA tone by EP4 modulating Kv channels with different oxygen tension between preterm and term. International Journal of Cardiology, 2011; 147(1) 58-65.

[105] McNamara, D.M., et al. Controlled trial of intravenous immune globulin in recent-onset dilated cardiomyopathy. Circulation, 2001; 103(18) 2254-9.

[106] Schultheiss, H.P., Kuhl, U., and Cooper, L.T. The management of myocarditis. European Heart Journal, 2011; 32(21) 2616-25.

[107] Tanaka, A., et al. An angiotensin II receptor antagonist reduces myocardial damage in an animal model of myocarditis. Circulation, 1994; 90(4) 2051-5.

[108] Sliwa, K., et al. Randomised investigation of effects of pentoxifylline on left-ventricular performance in idiopathic dilated cardiomyopathy. Lancet, 1998; 351(9109) 1091-3.

[109] Saura, M., et al. An antiviral mechanism of nitric oxide: inhibition of a viral protease. Immunity, 1999; 10(1) 21-8.

[110] Padalko, E., et al. Peroxynitrite inhibition of Coxsackievirus infection by prevention of viral RNA entry. Proceedings of the National Academy of Sciences of the United States of America, 2004; 101(32) 11731-6.

[111] Zell, R., et al. Nitric oxide donors inhibit the coxsackievirus B3 proteinases 2A and 3C in vitro, virus production in cells, and signs of myocarditis in virus-infected mice. Medical Microbiology and Immunology, 2004; 193(2-3) 91-100.

[112] Gwathmey, K., Balogun, R.A., and Burns, T. Neurologic indications for therapeutic plasma exchange: an update. Journal of Clinical Apheresis, 2011; 26(5) 261-8.

[113] Bulut, D., et al. Effects of immunoadsorption on endothelial function, circulating endothelial progenitor cells and circulating microparticles in patients with inflammatory dilated cardiomyopathy. Clinical Research in Cardiology, 2011; 100(7) 603-10.

[114] Sidwell, R.W., Robins, R.K., and Hillyard, I.W. Ribavirin: an antiviral agent. Pharmacology and Therapeutics, 1979; 6(1) 123-46.

[115] Kishimoto, C., Crumpacker, C.S., and Abelmann, W.H. Ribavirin treatment of murine coxsackievirus B3 myocarditis with analyses of lymphocyte subsets. Journal of the American College of Cardiology, 1988; 12(5) 1334-41.

[116] Harki, D.A., et al. Synthesis and antiviral activity of 5-substituted cytidine analogues: identification of a potent inhibitor of viral RNA-dependent RNA polymerases. Journal of Medicinal Chemistry, 2006; 49(21) 6166-9.

[117] Badorff, C., et al. Nitric oxide inhibits dystrophin proteolysis by coxsackieviral protease 2A through S-nitrosylation: A protective mechanism against enteroviral cardiomyopathy. Circulation, 2000; 102(18) 2276-81.

[118] Gluck, B., et al. Cardioprotective effect of NO-metoprolol in murine coxsackievirus B3-induced myocarditis. Journal of Medical Virology, 2010; 82(12) 2043-52.

[119] Ding, Y., et al. Influence of cinnamaldehyde on viral myocarditis in mice. American Journal of the Medical Sciences, 2010; 340(2) 114-20.

[120] Yun, S.H., et al. Antiviral activity of coxsackievirus B3 3C protease inhibitor in experimental murine myocarditis. Journal of Infectious Diseases, 2012; 205(3) 491-7.

[121] Fairweather, D., et al. Interferon-gamma protects against chronic viral myocarditis by reducing mast cell degranulation, fibrosis, and the profibrotic cytokines transforming growth factor-beta 1, interleukin-1 beta, and interleukin-4 in the heart. American Journal of Pathology, 2004; 165(6) 1883-94.

[122] Henke, A., et al. Direct interferon-gamma-mediated protection caused by a recombinant coxsackievirus B3. Virology, 2003; 315(2) 335-44.

[123] Daliento, L., et al. Successful treatment of enterovirus-induced myocarditis with interferon-alpha. Journal of Heart and Lung Transplantation, 2003; 22(2) 214-7.

[124] Zimmermann, O., et al. Interferon beta-1b therapy in chronic viral dilated cardiomyopathy--is there a role for specific therapy? Journal of Cardiac Failure, 2010; 16(4) 348-56.

[125] Kuhl, U., et al. Interferon-beta treatment eliminates cardiotropic viruses and improves left ventricular function in patients with myocardial persistence of viral genomes and left ventricular dysfunction. Circulation, 2003; 107(22) 2793-8.

[126] Wang, Y.X., et al. Antiviral and myocyte protective effects of murine interferon-beta and -{alpha}2 in coxsackievirus B3-induced myocarditis and epicarditis in Balb/c mice. American Journal of Physiology. Heart and Circulatory Physiology, 2007; 293(1) H69-76.

[127] Frustaci, A., Russo, M.A., and Chimenti, C. Randomized study on the efficacy of immunosuppressive therapy in patients with virus-negative inflammatory cardiomyopathy: the TIMIC study. European Heart Journal, 2009; 30(16) 1995-2002.

[128] Padalko, E., et al. The interferon inducer ampligen [poly(I)-poly(C12U)] markedly protects mice against coxsackie B3 virus-induced myocarditis. Antimicrobial Agents and Chemotherapy, 2004; 48(1) 267-74.

[129] Yu, Z., et al. Oral administration of interferon-alpha2b-transformed Bifidobacterium longum protects BALB/c mice against coxsackievirus B3-induced myocarditis. Virology Journal, 2011; 8 525.

[130] Ahn, J., et al. Antiviral effects of small interfering RNA simultaneously inducing RNA interference and type 1 interferon in coxsackievirus myocarditis. Antimicrobial Agents and Chemotherapy, 2012; 56(7) 3516-23.

[131] Yanagawa, B., et al. Coxsackievirus B3-associated myocardial pathology and viral load reduced by recombinant soluble human decay-accelerating factor in mice. Laboratory Investigation, 2003; 83(1) 75-85.

[132] Dorner, A., et al. Alternatively spliced soluble coxsackie-adenovirus receptors inhibit coxsackievirus infection. Journal of Biological Chemistry, 2004; 279(18) 18497-503.

[133] Lim, B.K., et al. Virus receptor trap neutralizes coxsackievirus in experimental murine viral myocarditis. Cardiovascular Research, 2006; 71(3) 517-26.

[134] Goodfellow, I.G., et al. Inhibition of coxsackie B virus infection by soluble forms of its receptors: binding affinities, altered particle formation, and competition with cellular receptors. Journal of Virology, 2005; 79(18) 12016-24.

[135] Dorner, A., et al. Treatment of coxsackievirus-B3-infected BALB/c mice with the soluble coxsackie adenovirus receptor CAR4/7 aggravates cardiac injury. Journal of Molecular Medicine, 2006; 84(10) 842-51.

[136] Demain, A.L. and Zhang, L. Natural Products and Drug Discovery. in: Zhang L, D.A. (ed.) Natural Products: Drug Discovery and Therapeutics Medicines. Totowa, NJ: Humana Press; 2005. p3-32.

[137] Zhang, L. Integrated Approaches for Discovering Novel Drugs From Microbial Natural Products. in: Zhang, L. and Demain, A.L. (ed.) Natural Products: Drug Discovery and Therapeutics Medicines. Totowa, NJ: Humana Press; 2005. p33-56.

[138] Zhang, L., et al. High-throughput synergy screening identifies microbial metabolites as combination agents for the treatment of fungal infections. Proceedings of the National Academy of Sciences of the United States of America, 2007; 104(11) 4606-11.

[139] Song, F., et al. Trichodermaketones A-D and 7-O-methylkoninginin D from the marine fungus Trichoderma koningii. Journal of Natural Products, 2010; 73(5) 806-10.

[140] Ashforth, E.J., et al. Bioprospecting for antituberculosis leads from microbial metabolites. Natural Product Reports, 2010; 27(11) 1709-19.

[141] Liu, Z.L., et al. Chinese herbal medicines for hypercholesterolemia. Cochrane Database of Systematic Reviews, 2011(7) CD008305.

[142] Zhang, Y., et al. Astragaloside IV exerts antiviral effects against coxsackievirus B3 by upregulating interferon-gamma. Journal of Cardiovascular Pharmacology, 2006; 47(2) 190-5.

[143] Chen, P., et al. Astragaloside IV attenuates myocardial fibrosis by inhibiting TGF-beta1 signaling in coxsackievirus B3-induced cardiomyopathy. European Journal of Pharmacology, 2011; 658(2-3) 168-74.

[144] Zhang, Y., et al. Antiviral effects of sophoridine against coxsackievirus B3 and its pharmacokinetics in rats. Life Sciences, 2006; 78(17) 1998-2005.

[145] Wang, Y.F., et al. Phyllaemblicin B inhibits Coxsackie virus B3 induced apoptosis and myocarditis. Antiviral Research, 2009; 84(2) 150-8.

[146] Mohsin, S., et al. Empowering adult stem cells for myocardial regeneration. Circulation Research, 2011; 109(12) 1415-28.

[147] Soler-Botija, C., Bago, J.R., and Bayes-Genis, A. A bird's-eye view of cell therapy and tissue engineering for cardiac regeneration. Annals of the New York Academy of Sciences, 2012; 1254 57-65.

[148] Alcon, A., Cagavi Bozkulak, E., and Qyang, Y. Regenerating functional heart tissue for myocardial repair. Cellular and Molecular Life Sciences, 2012; 69(16) 2635-56.

[149] Nagaya, N., et al. Transplantation of mesenchymal stem cells improves cardiac function in a rat model of dilated cardiomyopathy. Circulation, 2005; 112(8) 1128-35.

[150] Li, J.H., Zhang, N., and Wang, J.A. Improved anti-apoptotic and anti-remodeling potency of bone marrow mesenchymal stem cells by anoxic pre-conditioning in diabetic cardiomyopathy. Journal of Endocrinological Investigation, 2008; 31(2) 103-10.

[151] Van Linthout, S., et al. Mesenchymal stem cells improve murine acute coxsackievirus B3-induced myocarditis. European Heart Journal, 2011; 32(17) 2168-78.

[152] Miteva, K., et al. Human cardiac-derived adherent proliferating cells reduce murine acute Coxsackievirus B3-induced myocarditis. PLoS ONE, 2011; 6(12) e28513.

[153] Zhang, F., et al. Cellular cardiomyoplasty for a patient with heart failure. Cardiovascular Radiation Medicine, 2003; 4(1) 43-6.

[154] Siminiak, T., et al. Autologous skeletal myoblast transplantation for the treatment of postinfarction myocardial injury: phase I clinical study with 12 months of follow-up. American Heart Journal, 2004; 148(3) 531-7.

[155] Stamm, C., et al. Autologous bone-marrow stem-cell transplantation for myocardial regeneration. Lancet, 2003; 361(9351) 45-6.

[156] Chachques, J.C., et al. Cellular cardiomyoplasty: clinical application. Annals of Thoracic Surgery, 2004; 77(3) 1121-30.